"In Arizona, you can hike through deep canyons, listening to the music of a desert creek and the soft rustle of cottonwood leaves. You can walk the crest of a forested mountain range through cool sylvan glades, observing the shimmering heat of the desert vistas far below through trembling aspen leaves."

—-Introduction

"You can't miss Showerbath Spring, which pours from an overhanging mass of travertine rock on the left side of Kanab Creek. As its name implies, the spring makes a fine, cool shower on a warm day."

— Kanab Canyon Loop, Trip 5

"This is an especially scenic and remote loop around Powell Plateau along the Colorado River. Several permanent streams grace the route, including Thunder River, Shinumo Creek, and White Creek. You'll spend days h...

banks, or along the tops of cliffs a few hundred fee...

—Powell Plateau Loo...

"Backpackers in the Blue Range have the exciting p... ...y of seeing or hearing a wolf. In 1998, Mexican Gray Wolves were reintroduced in the Apache National Forest as part of a program to rescue the wolves from the edge of extinction. Currently, about two dozen wolves range freely in the Gila and Apache national forests."

—KP-Grant Creek Loop, Trip 11

"The Strayhorse Loop includes a unique section of hiking along the Blue River, and has the flavor of hiking in Arizona before the recreation explosion, when trailheads were rarely marked, backcountry trails were almost unused, and trail signs often missing."

—Strayhorse Loop, Trip 12

"As you climb, a panoramic view of Canyon Lake and the rugged terrain around it opens behind you; don't forget to take a break and look back! You're hiking through classic Sonoran desert, and such distinctive plants as the giant saguaro cactus and green-barked palo verde trees dominate the landscape."

—La Barge-Boulder Canyon Loop, Trip 19

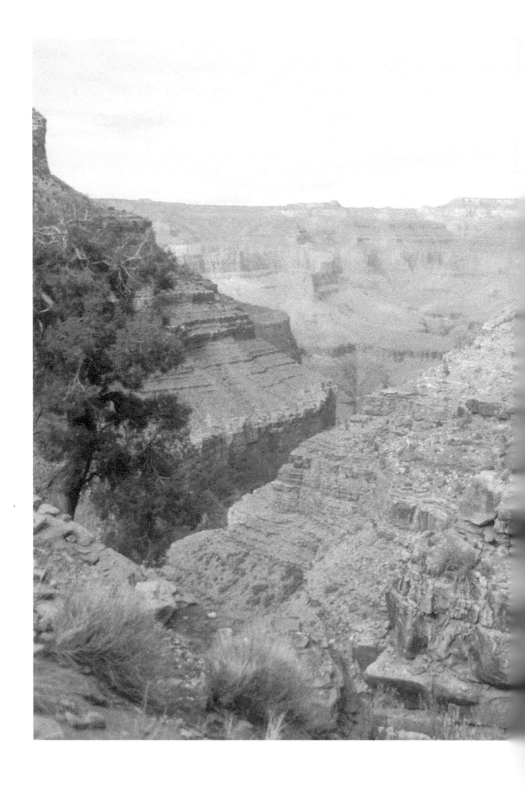

Backpacking
ARIZONA

From
Deep Canyons
to Sky Islands

Bruce Grubbs

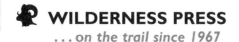

WILDERNESS PRESS
. . . on the trail since 1967

Backpacking Arizona

1ST EDITION September 2003
  3rd printing 2012

Copyright © 2003 by Bruce Grubbs

Front cover photo © 2003 by Tom Till
Back cover photo © 2003 by Bruce Grubbs
Interior photos, except where noted, by Bruce Grubbs
Maps: Bruce Grubbs
Cover design: Jaan Hitt
Book design: Wilsted & Taylor and Jaan Hitt
Book editor: Peter Hines

ISBN 978-0-89997-324-1

Manufactured in the United States of America

Published by: **Wilderness Press**
               Keen Communications
               P.O. Box 43673
               Birmingham, AL 35243
               (800) 443-7227; FAX (205) 326-1012
               info@wildernesspress.com
               www.wildernesspress.com

Visit our website for a complete listing of our books and for ordering information.

Distributed by Publishers Group West

Cover photos: *Hiking the Tonto Plateau in Grand Canyon* (front, top); *San Francisco
               Peaks* (front, bottom left); *Pine Mountain* (front, bottom center);
               Courthouse Rock, Eagletail Mountains (front, bottom right); *Mount
               Baldy Loop* (back, top); *Midnight Mesa Loop* (back, bottom)

Frontispiece: © 2003, Roslyn Bullas, *Hermit Trail, Grand Canyon National Park*

Acknowledgments

I'd like to extend a warm thanks to all my backpacking companions over the years. Special thanks to Duart Martin, whose encouragement and support made this book possible.

Safety Notice

Although backpacking is probably safer than the drive to the trailhead, there is some risk involved. By its very nature, backpacking involves travel in remote wilderness areas where help may be days away. Anyone planning to do the trips described in this book must plan to be completely self-sufficient while in the backcountry. At least one member of the party should be experienced, and all group members should be properly equipped and fit for wilderness travel. Because trail conditions, weather, and hiker abilities all vary considerably, the author and the publisher cannot assume responsibility for the safety of anyone who takes these hikes. Backcountry safety is mostly a matter of common sense and being aware of your abilities and limitations. All water sources mentioned in the hike descriptions, except for the Bright Angel Trail option on the Nankoweap–Bright Angel Loop, are untreated and must be purified before use.

Tell us what you really think Something unclear, outdated, or just plain wrong in this book? Have a good suggestion for making it better? We welcome reader feedback on all our publications. If we use your suggestion, we'll send you a free book. Please email comments to: update@wildernesspress.com

To my parents, who got me into the wilderness.

Featured Trips Overview Map

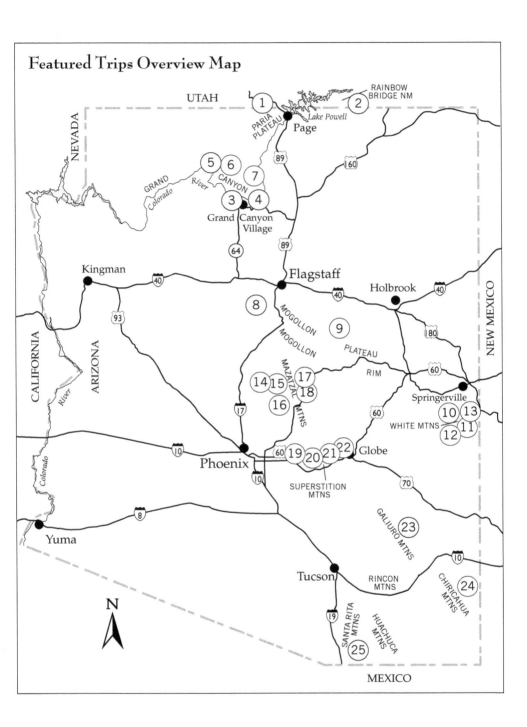

Contents

RIM COUNTRY

SKY ISLANDS

Map Legend

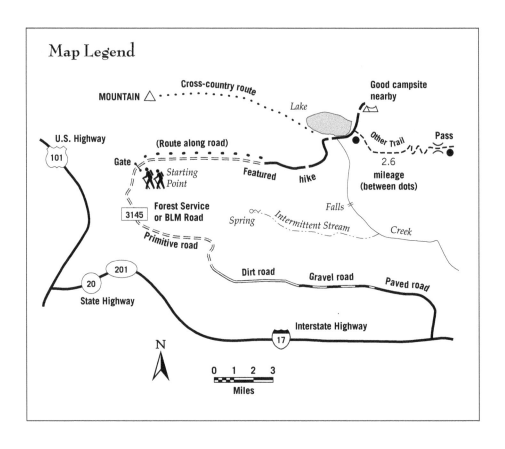

Featured Trips Summary Chart

TRIP	SCENERY	SOLITUDE	DIFFICULTY	MILES	ELEVATION GAIN	DAYS
Best in spring and fall						
1 Paria Canyon	10	3	4	37.0	0	4
2 Rainbow Bridge	9	8	7	23.9	4740	3
3 South Bass Trail to Hermit Trail	10	7	6	42.7	5970	5
4 Tanner Trail to Kaibab Trail	10	6	7	47.5	7580	6
5 Kanab Canyon Loop	10	9	9	52.2	5570	7
7 Nankoweap-Bright Angel Loop	10	10	10	82.2	16,830	11
8 Sycamore Canyon	8	7	7	55.7	6120	6
9 Historic Canyon Loop	7	6	4	21.8	2860	3
12 Strayhorse Loop	7	9	7	33.8	4240	5
14 Wet Bottom Loop	8	7	7	42.6	7680	5
15 Midnight Mesa Loop	8	9	7	40.6	7650	6
16 Deadman Creek Loop	7	9	8	57.7	11,510	7
17 Y Bar-Rock Creek Loop	7	7	6	19.8	5190	2
18 Deer Creek-Y Bar Loop	8	8	6	26.7	4950	3
23 Holdout Spring Loop	7	9	6	25.0	5520	3
Best in summer and fall						
10 Mount Baldy Loop	9	5	6	15.8	2720	2
11 KP-Grant Creek Loop	7	7	6	34.6	4440	4
13 WS Mountain Loop	7	8	6	23.8	4220	3
24 Chiricahua Crest	8	3	3	15.2	1890	2
25 Santa Rita Crest	8	3	4	13.3	4030	2
Best in fall						
6 Powell Plateau Loop	10	10	10	54.6	7250	9
Best in fall, winter, and spring						
19 La Barge-Boulder Canyon Loop	8	4	6	26.2	3840	3
20 Red Tanks Divide Loop	8	6	5	26.2	4360	3
21 Fish Creek Loop	8	6	5	21.7	3160	3
22 Campaign Creek Loop	7	7	5	29.9	5820	3

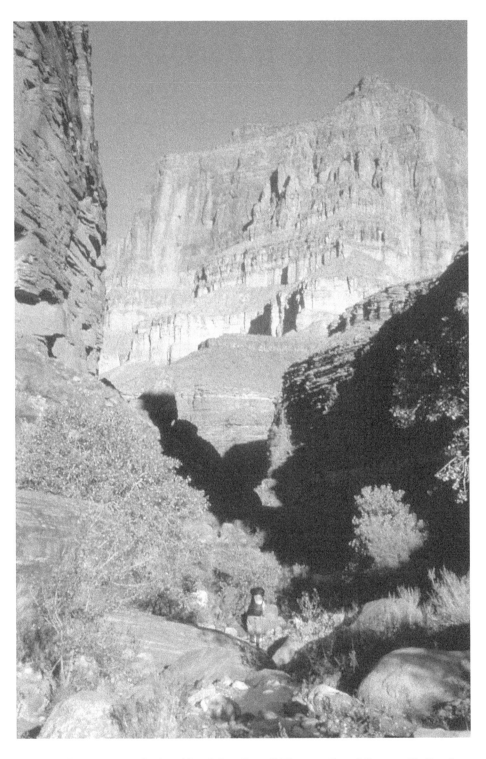

Cross-country backpacking below Powell Plateau, Grand Canyon National Park, Trip 6

Introduction

This book is a backpacker's guide to hiking in Arizona. While many hiking guides cover Arizona, all of them emphasize day hikes. *Backpacking Arizona* primarily describes backpacking trips of three to six days, although a few overnight hikes and several trips of a week or longer are included.

Experienced local hikers know that backpacking is one of the best ways to enjoy Arizona's incredible diversity and beauty. Carrying all you need to live comfortably in the wilderness for days at a time gives the hiker a satisfying feeling of self-sufficiency. Such a "house on your back" enables the backpacker to travel deep into the backcountry, far beyond the reach of hikers limited to a single day. In all but a few places, Arizona backpackers are free to camp nearly anywhere, at sites whose pristine beauty is beyond the imagination of the legions of vehicle recreationists who camp in a few designated campgrounds or heavily overused roadside campsites. Backpacking loads don't have to be heavy, although some trips do require you to carry heavy water loads. Modern lightweight equipment greatly reduces the load on your back, and there's a large selection of high-tech packs available that make carrying your gear surprisingly comfortable.

In Arizona, you can hike through deep canyons, listening to the music of a desert creek and the soft rustle of cottonwood leaves. You can walk the crest of a forested mountain range through cool sylvan glades, observing the shimmering heat of the desert vistas far below through the trembling aspen leaves. You can spend ten days or more wandering the depths of a great canyon system, where even human footprints are rare. You can loop from cactus-studded desert to forested mountains and back to the desert, without seeing another person for days on end, and never be more than fifty miles from the state's largest city.

The backpacking trips described in this book are necessarily a reflection of my experience. While I have attempted to present a selection of the best backpack trips in the state, no roomful of Arizona backpackers could ever agree on such a list. You'll notice right away that the majority of trips are loops. In my opinion, loops are the best backpack trips. Loops eliminate the need for a second vehicle for a car shuttle, and they make the most of your valuable backpacking vacation time. The last thing a backpacker wants to do is spend a day bouncing over dusty roads instead of walking gently through the backcountry. You'll find only two out-and-back hikes in this book, both through country so unique and beautiful that you'll not mind seeing the same scenery twice. Of course, there are some great backpack trips that just can't be done as loops. These trips use trailheads that are as close together as possible, or have commercial shuttle services or public transit available.

Guidebook writers face an unpleasant dilemma. Such books tend to attract large crowds of people to the described areas. On the other hand, without people who have experienced and appreciated the backcountry, wilderness will have no defenders. Long ago I decided that the risks of large invasions are more than offset by the larger voice they create for the defense of wild country. And make no mistake—the forces of development, driven by people who honestly feel that every corner of the planet should be exploited for human use and corporate profit, are relentless. Only an aware citizenry can stand up for places and creatures that cannot speak for themselves.

That said, every backpacker shares the responsibility to leave no trace of his or her presence. Arizona wilderness is dry, plants are slow growing, and litter lasts for centuries. Adopt the United States Forest Service's "Pack it in, pack it out" slogan. Simply put, if you carried it in, you can carry it out. Never bury or burn any sort of trash. Animals dig up food scraps, and man-made materials such as plastics degrade slowly or not at all. Most backcountry litter is accidental, and we can all help by packing out a bit of litter on every trip.

When following a trail, stay on it and do not cut switchbacks. Taking shortcuts greatly increases erosion and trail maintenance

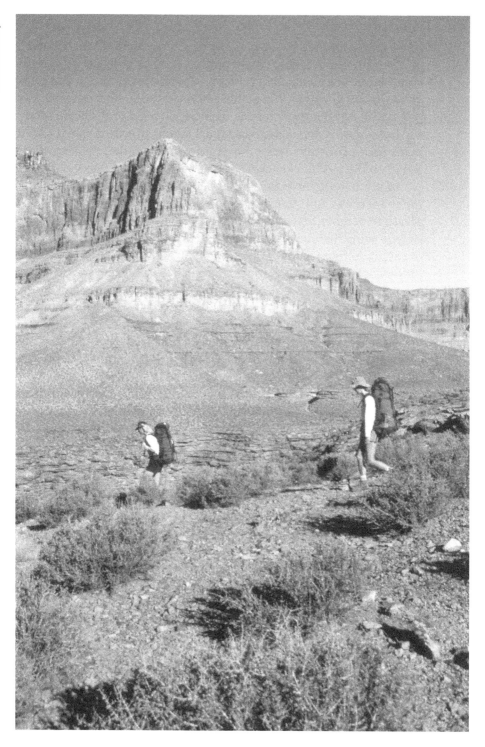

Desert scenery along the Tonto Plateau

costs, and you'll always expend more energy than if you followed on the trail. When hiking cross-country, avoid fragile terrain such as cryptobiotic soil as much as possible. Cryptobiotic soil is a thin crust of cooperating plants that forms in desert areas, and especially in pinyon pine and juniper forests. The fragile crust protects the sandy soil from erosion and takes many years to reform once crushed. Don't build rock cairns to mark your cross-country route. Such markers diminish the next backpacker's experience and aren't necessary.

Many hikers, including some backpackers, enjoy experiencing the wilderness with their four-footed companions. I like dogs, but please remember that not every backpacker does, and no one appreciates having their backcountry experience marred by dogs that bark or run up to them in an intimidating way. Also, dogs are a menacing presence to most wildlife, and certain predators will attempt to entice your dog away from you. Dogs are not allowed on trails or in the backcountry of most national parks. In national forests, dogs must be kept under control at all times, either by voice command or leash. If your dog runs up to other backpackers, chases wildlife, and does not come instantly at your command, it is not under control and must be on a leash or left at home.

Camping causes the most damage to the backcountry, but good equipment and technique can alleviate nearly all impact. The use of high-quality shelters (tarps, bivi sacks, or tents), sleeping bags, and sleeping pads completely eliminate the need to "improve" a site for comfort, warmth, or safety. The worst campsite "improvement" is a campfire ring. Campfire scars, often full of unburnable trash, mar far too many beautiful places. Never build campfires, except in an emergency. If you have a lightweight, warm sleeping bag and jacket, you'll stay warmer than you would huddling around a campfire. You'll also get to enjoy the wider worlds of night sounds, smells, and sky instead of a small circle of smoky light.

If you do build a campfire, *never* leave it unattended. Before leaving camp, *put your fire out completely.* To do this, mix the coals with water repeatedly until there is no heat or smoke, then feel the ashes with your hands to make certain it is out. If you can't do this, your fire is not out. If you don't have enough water, use dirt. This accomplishes the same thing as water but takes longer. Never leave a campfire or bury it in dirt. Campfires can easily escape from under a layer of dirt. Abandoned campfires have caused some of Arizona's

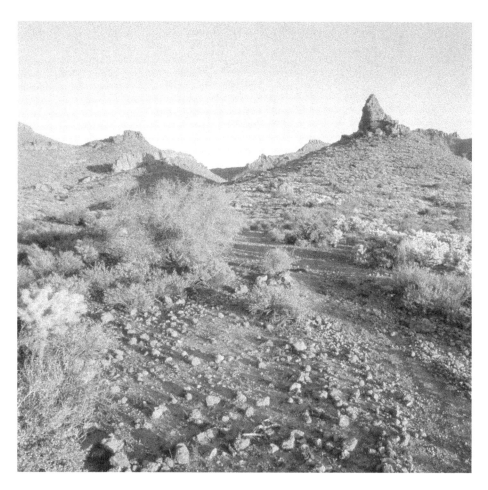

Superstition Wilderness

worst wildfires, including one that burned the entire Four Peaks Wilderness in 1966: more than 60,000 acres were burned. Smoking is another common cause of wildfires. In the national forests, it is illegal to smoke while traveling along the trails or cross-country. Smokers are required to stop and clear a two-foot circle to bare earth, and then make certain that all smoking materials are extinguished before leaving.

Once away from facilities, most people have little knowledge of basic human sanitation. Fortunately, the word has spread among backpackers and most seem to know what to do, but Arizona's dry climate warrants special consideration. Since springs, water pockets,

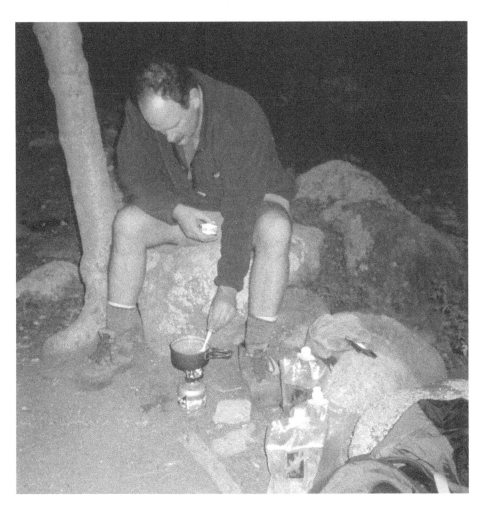

Camp at Fish Creek, Superstition Wilderness, Trip 21

creeks, and rivers are especially precious here, make an extra effort to answer the call of nature at least one hundred yards from any water, preferably further. The normal practice of digging a small "cat hole" for your waste works well, except in barren, sandy soil. Try to find a spot where the soil is rich in organic material, if possible. Most rangers and land managers now recommend that all used toilet paper should be carried out. It is slow to degrade in the dry climate, and burning it poses an unacceptable fire hazard much of the year. Pack it out in doubled zipper plastic bags, and add a bit of baking soda to control the odor.

HOW TO USE THIS GUIDE

Scenery

This is the author's opinion of the trip's overall scenic beauty, on a scale of 1 (ugly) to 10 (unsurpassed). Obviously this rating is highly subjective and dependent on the author's tastes. Remember that all of the trips have been carefully selected from a plethora of candidates, and all of them are scenic. Some are more scenic than others, so use this rating as a guide to relative scenic qualities.

Solitude

Most backpackers prize solitude. With this rating, you can get an idea of the degree of solitude to expect, from 1 (you'll be elbowing your way through crowds) to 10 (you won't see a soul, even on holiday weekends). Remember that even popular, crowded areas may be very lonely during mid-week and off-season. On the other hand, a quiet, remote area may be invaded by a large group sponsored by an organization.

Difficulty

This is another subjective rating that is intended to rate a trip's difficulty in relation to other backpack trips. Dayhikers unaccustomed to carrying heavy loads will probably find the easiest of these trips to be strenuous, and couch potato non-hikers will have a very tough time. If you have some backpacking experience, expect a 1 to be a straightforward hike on good trails. At the other extreme, you'll find that a 10 will probably have such obstacles as serious cross-country walking, tedious bushwhacking, difficult navigation, scarce water sources, and possible rock scrambling where packs may have to be hauled and some group members may want a belay. Backpackers attempting these most difficult trips should be fit, and at least one member of the party should be an experienced desert backpacker. Most trips in this book fall in between these limits.

Miles

This is basic mileage for the primary trip, with no side trips or options. Since official trail mileage varies widely in accuracy, the author measured the trip distance on 1:24000 scale U.S.G.S. topographic maps. Such map-derived distances tend to be slightly shorter than mileages measured with a trail wheel on the ground, but they are very consistent. A second mileage figure in parentheses below the primary number gives the total distance for the primary trip and all optional side trips described. Some of the loop trips have short-cut options that make the loop shorter. In this case the mileage in parentheses is less than the main loop mileage.

Elevation Gain

This number is an attempt to give the total elevation gain on the primary trip. It doesn't count minor ups and downs that are too small to show on a U.S.G.S. 1:24000 topographic map. A second number in parentheses shows the elevation gain or loss for the primary trip plus all optional side trips. Some of the loop trips have short-cut options. In this case the elevation gain in parentheses may be less than that of the main loop.

Days

One hiker's three-day backpack trip is another's dayhike! Nevertheless, this number is the author's recommendation, based on an average of 8 miles per day—a reasonable figure with a big pack in rough country. This figure is strongly influenced by the availability and spacing of water sources and good campsites. A second number in parentheses below the first gives the number of days required for the primary trip and all optional side trips in the description. Some of the loop hikes have an optional short cut, so the number of days required may be less.

Shuttle Mileage

If this number is 0, and the trip is a loop or an out-and-back hike, no shuttle is required. Otherwise, it shows the shortest driving distance between the beginning and ending trailheads. Remember to schedule enough time at the start and end of your hike to drive the shuttles. In a few areas, it's possible to hire a shuttle service that will drop you off at the starting trailhead, and then move your vehicle to the exit trailhead. Such services save a lot of time, and are listed under the contact information if available.

Maps

Each hike in the book includes an accurate sketch map to give you a general idea of the layout of the trip. You should also carry a topographic map covering the area. The most detailed maps are the U.S.G.S. 7.5 minute series of quadrangles, and the names of the maps covering the hike are always listed. If there is also an agency-issued or privately produced wilderness or recreation map covering the hike, its name is listed. These maps may have less terrain detail, but road and trail information is usually updated more often.

Season

The months listed are those in which the hike is possible, either snow-free for mountain hikes, or when the weather is reasonably cool for desert hikes.

Best

These months represent my opinion of when it's the best time to do the trip, a decision that is strongly influenced by the availability of water. Lesser factors include fall colors and wildflowers. Of course, most areas are at their most crowded during the best season; if solitude is your primary consideration, consider an off-season.

Water

The availability of water controls the planning of most Arizona backpack trips. This section lists all known springs, natural tanks, water pockets, and streams along the hike. I use the term "seasonal" to refer to creeks and springs that may have water only during the cool season and after wet weather. Very few water sources can be considered permanent.

> **Warning:** *Never depend on any single water source, and always have an alternate route, or even retreat, in mind if water sources are unexpectedly dry. All backcountry water should be purified before use, by chemical treatment, a water filter, or by boiling.*

Permits

Permits are required for some of the hikes in this book, and in certain areas only a limited number of backpackers are allowed. The permit requirements at the time of writing are described, but since the permit situation is changing rapidly on Arizona public lands, you should contact the land management agency before your trip for the latest information.

Rules

As land managers deal with increasing impact on the backcountry, they are often forced to impose special rules on hikers, such as campfire restrictions and group size limits. These rules are listed here, but do not include common backcountry rules such as the requirement to leave no trace, keep pets quiet and under control, and pack out everything you brought in.

Contact

This is the telephone number for the local land management agency that is responsible for the area of the hike. I also list a web site if a useful one is available. It's a good idea to call ahead and check on road and trail conditions, as well as permits and special requirements.

Highlights

This paragraph focuses on outstanding features such as the opportunity to see wildlife, exceptional views, narrow canyons, and other appealing attributes.

Problems

Unusual difficulties such as lack of water, poorly maintained trails, rough access roads, crowds, and other potential problems are listed here. Please remember that it's impossible for a book to list all the problems you may encounter in remote country.

How to Get There

This section describes the best access route from the nearest sizable town. Alternate routes are listed where appropriate, as is the route to the end of the hike if a shuttle is required. With a few exceptions, you'll need a vehicle to get to these backpack trips. While you can reach some trailheads on paved roads, most require travel on dirt roads that can be traversed by a normal vehicle. Some approaches do require high-clearance or four-wheel-drive vehicles. Because some trailheads are very remote, it's a good idea to carry extra water, food, and a change of clothes in your vehicle.

Description and Tips and Warnings

The detailed description includes clear navigation directions using natural landmarks and trail signs. Directions are given as left and right, and are backed up with the compass direction in parentheses. Although mileages between trail junctions are provided, the emphasis is placed on natural landmarks since mileage is difficult to measure in the backcountry and trail signs may be damaged or missing. Cross-country routes are described entirely by landmarks. *Tips* and *Warnings* are based on the author's experience and are embedded in the text to call your attention to things that may make your trip safer and more enjoyable.

Possible Itinerary

A suggested plan for the primary trip is listed after the description, based on the author's experience on the route. This may or may not include side trips. Side trips are clearly labeled as such. Treat itinerary as a starting point for your own trip planning, remembering that such things as water availability, trail conditions, and the fitness and experience level of the group will affect your final itinerary.

Optional Side Hikes, Shortcuts, and Alternate Routes

These are mentioned by name in the main description of each hike. An optional side hike offers you the chance to explore a feature, trail, or route off the main hike. These are usually done as out-and-back dayhikes. A shortcut is an optional route that shortens the length of the overall trip. An alternate route is an optional trail or route that is the same length or longer than the main trip.

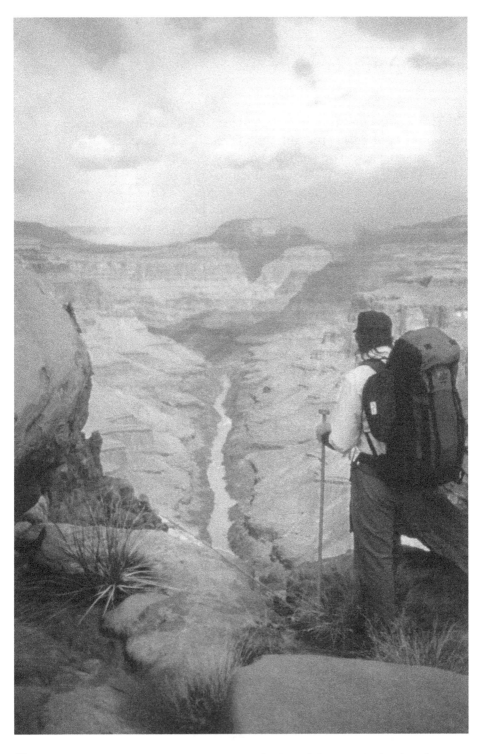

Conquistador Aisle from The Esplanade, Grand Canyon National Park

General Tips on
Backpacking in Arizona

WATER AND HEAT

Arizona is a desert state. The low deserts of the south and west sections of the state are dangerously hot in the summer. In this region, daily temperatures top 100°F from May through mid September, and readings of 110 or higher are common. The extreme heat creates extreme aridity, and the combination is frequently deadly to unprepared desert travelers. Even in the mountainous north-central and eastern sections of Arizona, where temperatures are moderated by elevations from 7000 to over 12,000 feet, the thin air remains dry much of the year.

Dehydration is a constant concern for the Arizona backpacker, and all trips must be planned around available water sources. Never depend on a single water source, such as a spring, creek, rock tank, or even a water cache you've placed yourself. Many springs and creeks are seasonal, flowing only during and immediately after the winter and summer wet season. Even permanent springs and streams may go dry during droughts. Carry enough water as you hike so that you can retreat to the last water source if a source is unexpectedly dry. Drink plenty of water, more than required to quench your thirst. Your body loses moisture insensibly in dry air, and you start to become dehydrated before you become thirsty. Electrolyte replacement drinks are very useful. Become familiar with the symptoms of heat exhaustion and sunstroke. Heat exhaustion is a debilitating condition brought on by heat and dehydration. If untreated, heat exhaustion can lead to sunstroke, caused by a complete loss of the body's ability to cool itself through sweating. Sunstroke is a serious medical emergency that is fatal if not treated immediately.

A useful skill to develop is the art of dry camping. When you have the freedom to camp well away from water sources, you'll find that it opens up many wonderful new campsites, such as ridges, saddles, and even mountaintops. (Of course, you should avoid camping on ridges and mountaintops during the thunderstorm season.) Planning a dry camp doesn't always mean carrying huge loads of water. A useful technique is to pick up water at a spring or creek late in the day and hike for another hour or two before camping. Arizona state law prohibits camping within 0.25 mile of a spring to allow wildlife access to water.

The best months to enjoy the lower elevation deserts are October through April. The days are commonly mild and clear, though temperatures may fall below freezing at night. Occasional winter rainstorms refresh the desert and bring out the late winter and spring flowers.

MOUNTAINS AND SNOW

At the other extreme, heavy snowfall is a frequent occurrence in the mountains above 6000 feet from December through March. Above 8000 feet, the snow pack is often several feet deep and makes backpacking impractical without snowshoes or skis. Snow falls in the fall and spring, but usually in small amounts that melt quickly. In the mountains, winter temperatures may drop well below zero, so the winter trekker must be prepared for the cold. For backpackers, the summer and autumn months are the best periods to enjoy the Arizona high country.

THE NORTH AMERICAN MONSOON

The hot, dry weather of May and June abruptly changes in July as a mass of moist tropical air typically moves in from the southeast. Skies, which have been clear for weeks, start to fill with puffy cumulus clouds by midmorning, and the afternoon often brings towering thunderstorms with strong gusty winds, heavy rain, hail, and lightning. Arizona lies at the northern limit of the North American Monsoon, which as the name implies is much more active south of the international border. The stormy weather follows a surge and break pattern, with active periods of several days or a week often followed by lulls when the moist air is pushed south of the state by minor weather disturbances. Still, take precautions during the monsoon. To avoid light-

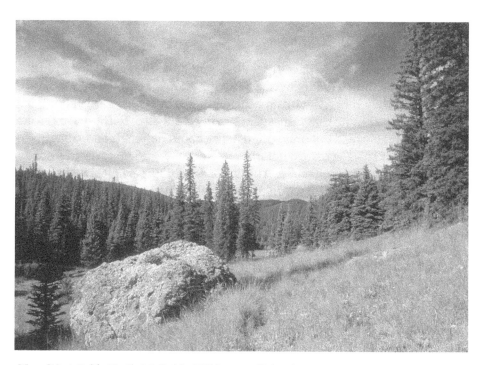

Near West Baldy Trail, Mt Baldy Wilderness, Trip 10

ning, plan to be off high ridges and peaks by midday. Because of the potential for floods, never camp or park a vehicle in dry washes or other drainages. Heavy rain may fall in the headwaters, miles from your location, and cause streams and dry washes to rise suddenly and without warning. If thunderstorms are building during the afternoon, plan to camp in a sheltered area, if possible. Thunderstorm gust fronts can produce winds of 60 miles per hour or more. Although most hailstorms are extremely local in nature, and seldom produce hailstones larger than 0.25 inch, larger hailstones do occur and can be dangerous to hikers caught in the open. That said, the summer rains are a delight. Monsoon mornings dawn clear and sweet, with mountain meadows misty with dew, and the afternoon clouds and rain bring welcome relief from the midday heat.

RATTLESNAKES, SCORPIONS, AND OTHER CRITTERS

Generally speaking, animals are a minor hazard in Arizona's backcountry. Rattlesnake bites are serious but uncommon among hikers, and they are rarely fatal. The best strategy is prevention. An awareness of rattlesnake habits allows you to avoid most unpleasant encounters. Rattlesnakes, like all snakes, are cold-blooded. They actively seek out surfaces that are about 80°F. In hot weather, rattlers will be in the shade; in cool weather, they'll be in the sun. In addition, they hibernate during the winter. If you see lizards about, it's safe to assume that rattlesnakes may be out also. Rattlesnakes strike extremely fast, but only to a distance about half their body length. To avoid rattlesnakes, do not place your hands and feet within reach of a possible hidden snake. This is especially important when passing near shady spots in warm weather, where it may be difficult to spot a snake trying to keep cool. Remember that rattlesnakes are probably more afraid of you than you are of them. Most will rattle and give you plenty of warning. When you do hear the unmistakable strident buzz of a nearby snake, stop immediately and locate the snake before moving carefully away. If a person does get bitten, the main hazard is infection from the deep fang wounds and tissue damage from the venom. When rattlesnakes strike defensively, the bite is often dry. The venom is usually reserved for hunting bites, where the hemotoxic venom not only kills mice and other small prey but also starts the digestive process. Most snakebite victims have been handling or teasing snakes. But if a member of your party does get bitten, keep the victim calm and at rest, and send other members of the party for a rescue.

Scorpions have been far more fatal to Arizonians over the years than snakes, though the victims are usually the very young or infirm. The most dangerous scorpion, the Arizona Bark Scorpion (*Centruroides excilicauda*), a small, straw-colored species found in the lowest desert areas, poses little threat to most healthy adults. Few of the hikes in this guide are located in these areas. The more common larger scorpions are found everywhere, but their sting is no more dangerous than a wasp sting. Again, knowing the critter's habits lets you avoid them. Scorpions are nocturnal, and during the day they lurk under rocks and logs. Always kick such objects with your boot before picking them up. Don't leave clothing or footwear outside your tent, or if you do, shake it out before wearing it.

Africanized bees have spread throughout Arizona, but are more common in the warmer, desert areas. They interbreed freely with the less aggressive, common honeybee, and only a lab analysis can tell them apart. Avoid all bees, especially if they are swarming. If attacked, drop your pack, run, do not swat at the bees, and protect

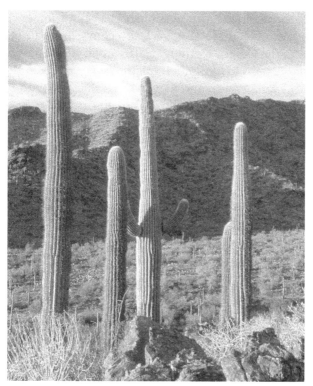

Saguaro cactus

your eyes. Africanized bees give up the chase after about half a mile. A vehicle or building is the best shelter, but in the backcountry, head for dense brush or vegetation, which confuses the bees. The sting of individual Africanized bees is no more dangerous than common bees—the danger lies in their aggressiveness.

Of course, anyone who is allergic to bee or insect stings should consult a doctor for treatment if stung. Hikers subject to severe reactions should carry antihistamines and an anti-sting kit.

CACTUS AND OTHER INTERESTING PLANTS

Cactus is found throughout the state, though only the Sonoran Desert of southwestern Arizona has the well-known giant saguaro cactus. Most cacti grow in isolated patches and are easily avoided. The cholla cactus propagates itself by growing easily dislodged joints.

The long, sharp spines have invisible barbs, so the joints cling tenaciously and are difficult to remove. Use a comb, or a pair of sticks, to pop them off the skin or clothing. Carry a pair of needlepoint tweezers to remove hard to see spines. Cactus spines are a serious hazard to air-filled sleeping pads, and they're often sharp enough to go right through a tent floor or groundsheet. Look the ground over very carefully before setting up your shelter. In poor light, it helps to sweep the ground with a light beam parallel to the ground.

Poison ivy is found along both perennial and seasonal streams at intermediate elevations in the mountains and canyon country. An organic acid in the sap causes the nasty skin reaction that many people suffer after contact. Washing immediately with water removes the water-soluble acid and lessens the chance of a reaction. Learn to recognize the distinctive, three-leafed, low-growing plant, and also the places where it's found, and you'll avoid problems. Remember that the acid gets on clothing, walking sticks, and dogs, as well as human skin.

PERMITS AND REGULATIONS

One of the great things about backpacking in Arizona is that the majority of wilderness areas do not require a permit. The major exceptions are the Grand Canyon National Park backcountry, which is highly regulated due to the overuse of a few popular areas, Saguaro National Park, and a few areas such as the Santa Catalina Mountains that are participating in the Federal Fee Demonstration Program. The current permit requirements and rules are listed with each hike, but since requirements may change, you should contact the managing agency before your trip for the latest information.

HUNTING SEASON

Check with the nearest Arizona Fish and Game office before your trip to find out if a hunt is being conducted in your area. The deer season during October and November brings out the most hunters, but the hunt takes place at different times across the state. Of course, all National Parks are closed to hunting.

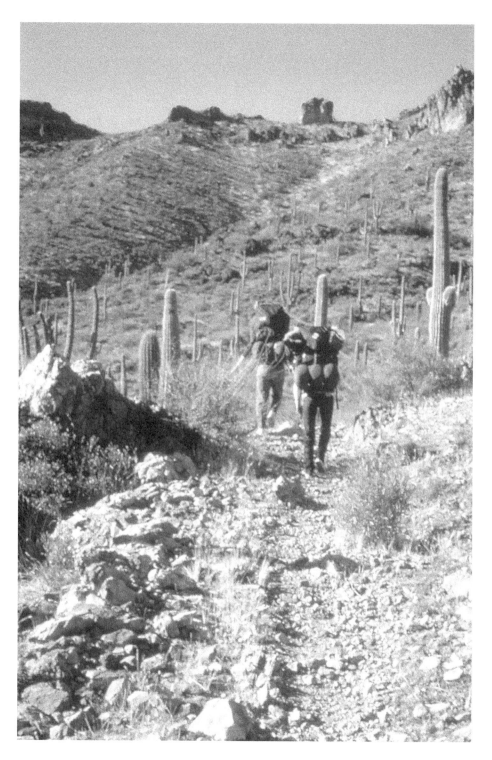

JF Trail, Superstition Mountains, Trip 21

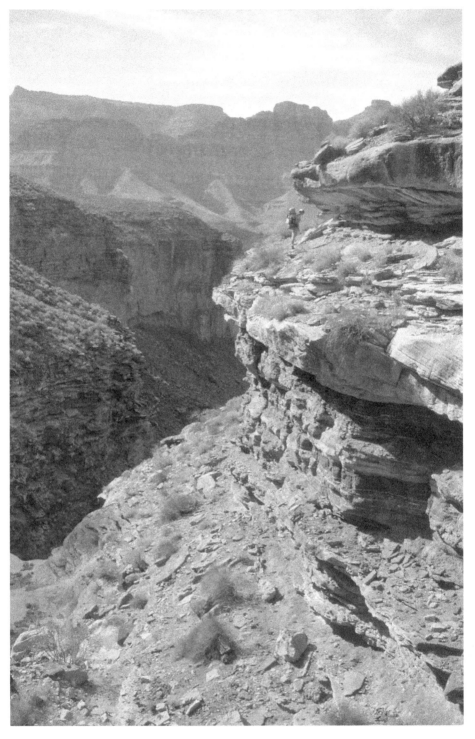

Tonto Trail, Grand Canyon National Park, Trip 3

Wild Areas of Arizona

This book is confined to those parts of the state most attractive to backpacking. The desert ranges in the southwestern quarter of the state are conspicuously missing from this book. While this region contains vast wilderness tracts, the region is not backpacker-friendly. The vast desert plains and low mountain ranges offer no trails, few defined cross-country routes, and almost no water. The backpack trips in this book focus on the areas that have a variety of terrain and enough water sources so that you do not have to carry punishing loads.

COLORADO PLATEAU

Slickrock Canyons

The Colorado Plateau is a varied landscape that covers approximately the northeastern third of Arizona, from the Mogollon Rim north and eastward into Utah, Colorado, and New Mexico. Sedimentary rocks such as sandstone, limestone, and shale, laid down in horizontal beds, form slickrock canyons and make up the bulk of the plateau. The plateau is not a single, level surface, but a series of plateaus varying in elevation from 3000 to over 12,000 feet. One of the continent's largest rivers, the Colorado, drains the western Rocky Mountains and cuts through the Colorado Plateau, creating a series of deep canyons along its length. Many of the side drainages carve their own canyons in turn, so that the surface of the plateau is dissected by upwards of 10,000 canyons. Towering above these deep canyons are scattered volcanic mountains. Two of the featured hikes explore canyon systems on the plateau.

Grand Canyon

The Grand Canyon, or "the Canyon," as locals refer to it, is the Colorado River's master achievement. It is more than 260 miles long, up to 20 miles wide, and over a mile deep, but such numbers don't convey the canyon's uniqueness. A colorful variety of sedimentary, metamorphic, and volcanic rocks are exposed in the Grand Canyon. These not only make for good scenery, but their character determines the shape of the canyon and controls the very routes that humans may use.

The Grand Canyon is not just a single large canyon. It is a maze of side canyons and tributaries, towering buttes, temples, and mesas. Hidden here and there are perennial streams, springs, and secret grottos. Nearly the entire canyon is included in Grand Canyon National Park, and most of the park is wilderness. Units of the Kaibab National Forest flank the park to the north and south. Elevations range from 8900 feet along the fir and aspen forests of the North Rim to 1200 feet along the creosote bush-lined banks of the lower Colorado River.

Despite the crowds at the developed sections of the south and north rims, and the popularity of a few trails, most of the canyon backcountry sees no visitors in a typical year. The catch is that only about ten percent of the backcountry is accessible by trail. To explore the rest, you'll have to hike cross-country through some of the most demanding terrain on Earth. This guidebook contains both trail and cross-country hikes in the Canyon, so you can learn the terrain on trails, and then progress to cross-country when you are ready.

RIM COUNTRY

Mogollon Rim

The Mogollon (pronounced "mug-e-on") Rim, an escarpment towering 2000 feet above the country to the south, runs across the state from the west end of the Grand Canyon to the Mogollon Mountains in New Mexico. The Mogollon Rim, which reaches elevations of 9300 feet, separates the Colorado Plateau from the central mountains. Just north of the Mogollon Rim, the southern edge of the Colorado Plateau is named the Mogollon Plateau. The plateau consists of a series of northward-draining canyons and intervening ridges, all covered with the world's largest stand of ponderosa pines. Some of the canyons are protected as wilderness areas, and all of them form a

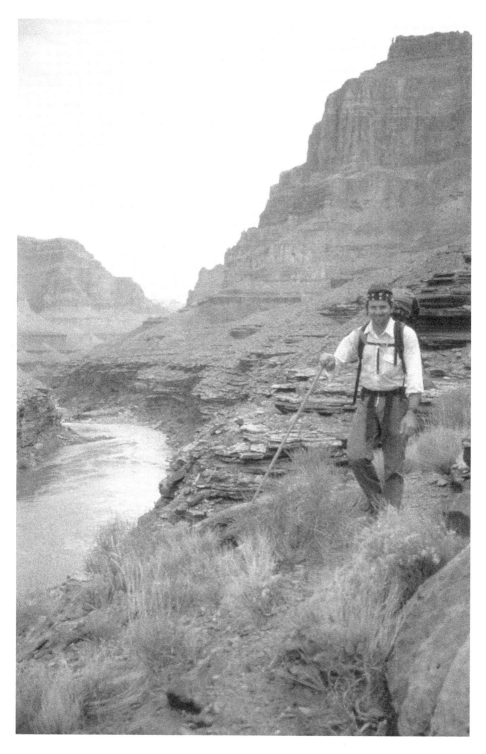

Cross-country backpacking below Powell Plateau, Grand Canyon National Park, Trip 6

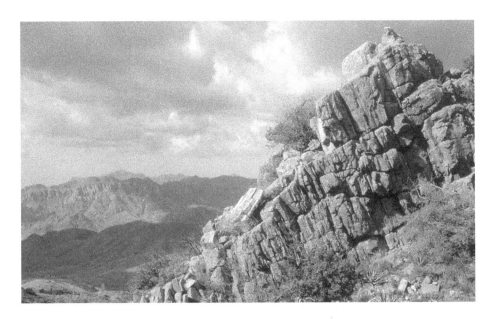

Near Iron Mountain, Superstition Wilderness

serious barrier to travel. Most of the rim country lies within the Kaibab, Coconino, and Apache-Sitgreaves National Forests.

White Mountains

Volcanic activity created the White Mountains near the eastern end of the Mogollon Rim. This area of high mesas and rounded summits lies partially in the White Mountain Apache Reservation, and partially within the Apache-Sitgreaves National Forest. Several wilderness areas in the White Mountain region protect heavily forested 11,000-foot mountains, as well as semidesert canyons at elevations below 5000 feet. The area of most appeal to backpackers is the Blue Range Primitive Area, known locally as the "Blue." This wild area straddles the Mogollon Rim east of the White Mountains.

The Mogollon Rim is split by the mile-deep canyon created by the Blue River, which drains south into the San Francisco River. West of the Blue River canyon the Mogollon Rim culminates at 9355-foot Blue Peak. 8000-foot mountains and plateaus rise along the Mogollon Rim east of the Blue River. Miles of seldom-used trails trace the Blue backcountry. In the 1930s, the Blue was one of the first wilderness areas protected by the U.S. Forest Service under the inspired leadership of Aldo Leopold. In 1964, Congress passed the Wilderness

Act, which included most of the Forest Service wilderness areas in the new National Wilderness Preservation System. The Forest Service designated the remaining administratively protected areas as primitive areas to distinguish them from Congressionally protected wilderness. In the years since, Congress has protected all the remaining primitive areas as wilderness areas, except one: the Blue. The administrative protection of the Blue by the U.S. Forest Service can be rescinded at any time. Even the small section of the Blue in New Mexico is protected as wilderness. Wilderness enthusiasts hope the Arizona section of the Blue will be added soon—it certainly deserves wilderness protection.

Central Mountains

All of Arizona south and west of the Mogollon Rim is part of the basin and range geologic province, in which small, separate north-south trending mountain ranges rise above intervening valleys. A rugged complex of mountains and deep valleys characterize the central mountains, the area immediately south of the Mogollon Rim. This vast area, mostly contained in the Tonto National Forest, contains a variety of terrain from desert canyons to forested plateaus and mountains.

Mazatzal Mountains

The Mazatzal Mountains, one of the largest and highest ranges in the central mountains, reaches 7903 feet at Mazatzal Peak. The Verde River, Arizona's only Wild and Scenic River and home to desert bald eagles, flows along the west side of the Mazatzal Wilderness Area. The crest of the Mazatzal Mountains is formed by a giant, tilted fault block of metamorphic rocks. This geology creates steep escarpments on the east, where water from the canyons drain into Tonto Creek. The west slopes are gentler, but are cut by deep, rugged canyons which empty into the Verde River at elevations around 2000 feet. The area is protected within the Mazatzal Wilderness, part of the Tonto National Forest. A network of trails covers the wilderness and provides the backpacker with a plethora of excellent wilderness trips from forested crest to desert plains.

Superstition Mountains

The Superstition Mountains, located at the southwestern edge of the central mountains, are mostly volcanic in character, the apparent remnants of a gigantic caldera. Local hikers fondly refer to the range as the "Sups." The western canyons and mountains of the Sups are part of the Sonoran Desert, and range from 2000 to 5000 feet in elevation. Desert shrubs, cactus, and grasslands are the primary vegetation in this western region. The eastern end of the Superstition Mountains features a metamorphic geology of largely granitic rocks. Elevations are higher in the eastern Sups, and the terrain is mostly covered with high desert grassland, chaparral brush, and pinyon pine and juniper woodland. A few pockets of stately ponderosa pines favor cool canyon bottoms and north slopes. Mound Mountain is the highest point in the Sups, at 6266 feet. The Superstition Wilderness Area encompasses nearly the entire range. Though relatively small, the wilderness is rugged and includes a thorough network of trails. This creates opportunities for a variety of backpack trips of several days.

SKY ISLANDS

Santa Catalina and Rincon Mountains

Arizona's basin and range country culminates in southeastern Arizona, where the mountain ranges reach as high as 10,700 feet. In the broad valleys separating the ranges, the Sonoran Desert of southwestern Arizona meets the Chihuahuan Desert of southern New Mexico, creating a mix of desert vegetation. But to the backpacker, the mountain ranges are of greatest interest. Crowned with forests of pine, fir, and aspen, and graced with springs and creeks, these isolated, lofty ranges are locally known as "sky islands." Nearly all the sky islands are part of the Coronado National Forest, and many are protected as wilderness areas. The 9157-foot Santa Catalina Mountains are the most accessible of the sky islands, just north of Tucson. Although a paved road leads to the top of the mountain, the western and southern sections are included in the Pusch Ridge Wilderness Area. The wilderness is a complex maze of deep canyons, creeks, and granite peaks, all laced by a network of trails. East of Tucson, Saguaro National Park contains the Rincon Mountains, an 8664-foot sky island. Both the Santa Catalina Mountains and the Rincon Mountains

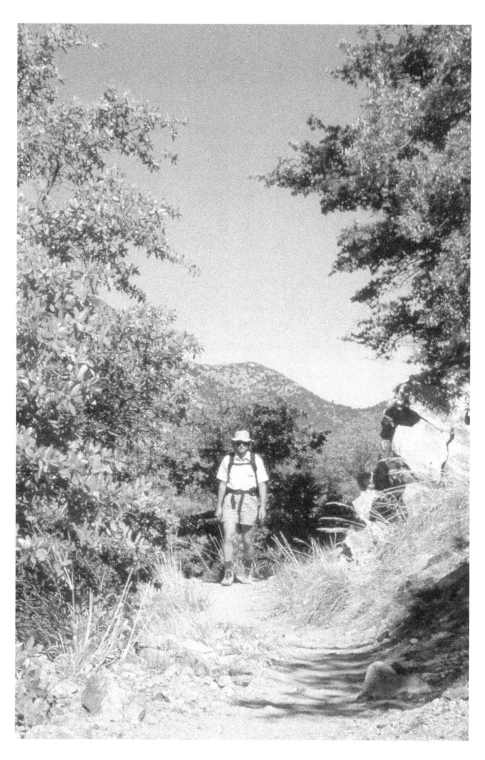

Along the Super Trail, Santa Rita Mountains, Trip 25

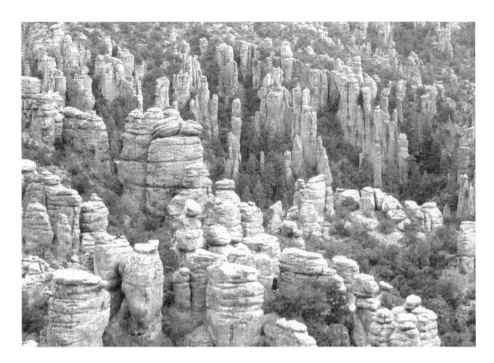

Pinnacles, Chiricahua Mountains

rise from 3000-foot desert valleys, and the vegetation ranges from classic saguaro cactus to fir, quaking aspen, and spruce.

Galiuro Mountains

Probably the least known sky island, the Galiuro Mountains top out at 7663-foot Bassett Peak. Vegetation is primarily high desert grassland and pinyon pine and juniper woodland. A few patches of ponderosa pines occur in protected valleys and on cooler north slopes. Deep canyons are the main feature of the range, and these are protected in the Galiuro Wilderness on the Coronado National Forest, and the Redfield Canyon Wilderness on Bureau of Land Management land. A network of little-used trails covers most of this remote sky island, and there are many possibilities for extended backpack trips into areas that rarely have visitors.

Chiricahua Mountains

The Chiricahua Mountains, another beautiful sky island, are in the southeast corner of the state, north of the town of Douglas. The crest of the Chiricahuas is a series of gentle, forested summits, culminating in 9759-foot Chiricahua Peak. Numerous canyons cut the flanks of the range, creating towering cliffs and dramatic vistas overlooking the 5000-foot valleys. The Chiricahua trail network provides many miles of enjoyable backpacking, from the Chihuahuan desert grasslands in the canyon bottoms, through chaparral brush and pinyon pine and juniper woodland, to graceful forests of Apache pine, quaking aspen, and Douglas-fir along the highest ridges.

Santa Rita Mountains

The prominent summit of 9453-foot Mount Wrightson crowns the Santa Rita Mountains south of Tucson. This unit of the Coronado National Forest is protected within the Mount Wrightson Wilderness. Because this sky island range is close to the Sierra Madre Mountains of northern Mexico, it forms a haven for rare birds normally seen only south of the international border. Several permanent streams further enhance the wildlife possibilities and contrast with the desert vegetation in the 3000- to 4000-foot valleys flanking the Santa Rita Mountains. Trails run the length of the crest and down the flanking ridges and canyons. Although the range is small, several rewarding overnight trips are possible in the Santa Rita Mountains.

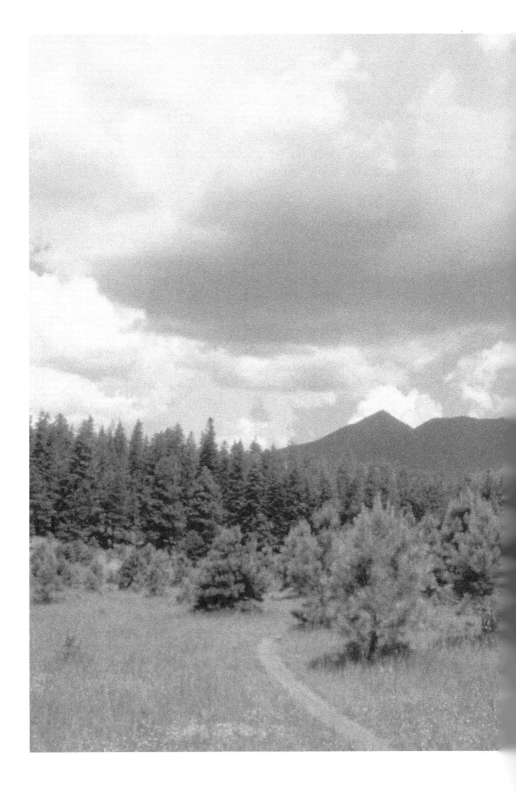

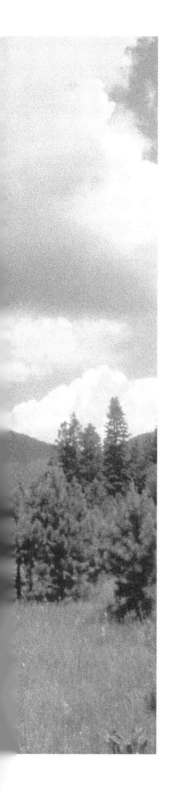

Featured Trips

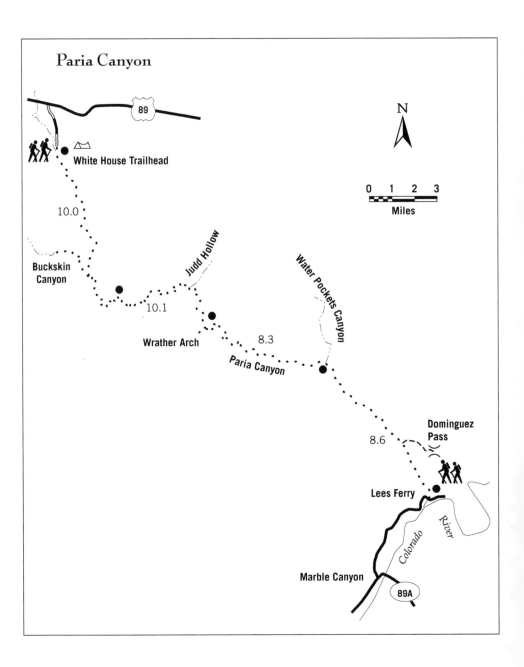

Paria Canyon

White House Trailhead

10.0

Buckskin
Canyon

Judd Hollow

10.1

Wrather Arch

8.3

Paria Canyon

Water Pockets Canyon

Dominguez
Pass

8.6

Lees Ferry

Colorado River

Marble Canyon

89A

N

0 1 2 3
Miles

1 Paria Canyon

RATINGS (1–10)			MILES	ELEVATION GAIN	DAYS	SHUTTLE MILEAGE
Scenery	Solitude	Difficulty	37.0	0	4	72
10	3	4	(43.0)	(2000)	(4)	

MAPS West Clark Bench, Bridger Point, Wrather Arch, Water Pockets, Ferry Swale, Lees Ferry U.S.G.S.

SEASON April–June, Mid-September through October.

BEST April–May, October.

WATER The Paria River generally flows below Buckskin Canyon, but the water is silty and must be filtered. You'll find several unnamed springs between miles 10 and 25.

PERMITS Required, and a reservation is recommended. Walk-in permits may be available, depending on demand, at the BLM Kanab Field Office or the Paria Information Station at the north trailhead, especially during the off-season (summer and winter).

RULES Campfires are not allowed and all toilet paper must be packed out.

CONTACT For information: Bureau of Land Management, 345 E. Riverside Dr. St. George, UT 84790, http://paria.az.blm.gov; for reservations: Arizona Strip Interpretive Association, 345 E. Riverside Dr., St. George, UT 84790, (435) 688-3246, ASFOWEB_Arizona@blm.gov

HIGHLIGHTS Starting just north of the Arizona border in southern Utah, this classic hike takes you through one of the most spectacular sandstone canyons in North America. Surprisingly, the hiking is reasonably easy—it's the only hike in this book with no elevation gain. A prime feature of this trip, the narrows of Paria Canyon, are 12 miles long, and average 20 to 30 feet wide and more than 500 feet deep. An optional side hike takes you into Buckskin Canyon, which is even narrower.

PROBLEMS Because Paria Canyon is popular, reservations are required for the limited number of permits available during the prime spring and fall seasons. A daily fee is charged for each person and each dog in the party. Although the Paria River is usually less than 1 foot deep, you'll cross it hundreds of times. You will need a pair of river sandals or other amphibious footwear. Conventional leather hiking boots will be ruined by a trip through Paria Canyon. A hiking stick is useful for maintaining your footing in the silty river.

Because a flash flood would be extremely dangerous in the narrows, and inconvenient elsewhere in the canyon, you must have a stable weather forecast before starting the trip. A storm in the Paria River's headwaters, completely out of your sight or hearing, can easily send a flash flood through the narrows. Hike the canyon north to south, as presented here, so that your weather forecast is as current as possible for the passage through the narrows from roughly mile 4 to 16. Summer weather can be extremely hot, and during the late fall and winter, the Paria River runs too high and cold to wade. A shuttle is necessary, so contact the BLM for a current list of commercial shuttle operators.

Warning: Before committing to the narrows, be certain you have a stable weather forecast for the Paria watershed, and that the actual weather matches the forecast.

HOW TO GET THERE To reach the starting point at White House Trailhead from Page, drive north 29 miles on U.S. 89 to the BLM ranger station and campground on the left (south) side of the highway. The end point of the trip at Lees Ferry on the Colorado River can be reached from Page by driving 23 miles south on U.S. 89 to Arizona 89A. Turn right (north), and continue 14 miles, across Navajo Bridge, and turn right (northeast) on the road to Lees Ferry, drive 5 miles and park in the west end of the long-term parking lot.

DESCRIPTION As you hike south from the White House Trailhead, the Paria River runs through an open valley, but within a couple of miles the canyon walls begin to close in, soon rising 200 feet above the Paria River bed. The narrows begin at about mile 4, where the canyon walls narrow to 20 to 50 feet. Paria Canyon is now over 400 feet deep. From here to about mile 12, there is no escape from rising water in the event of a flood, and no place to camp.

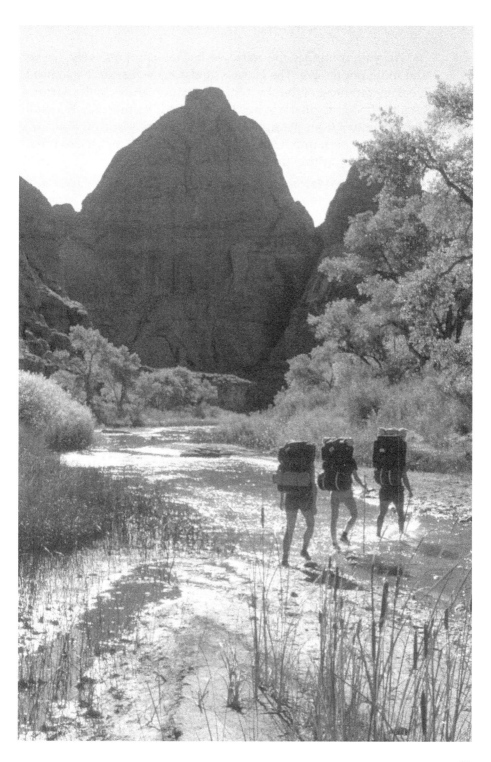

Backpackers in Paria Canyon

As you continue, the narrows become progressively deeper and more impressive. The Navajo sandstone walls curve overhead, blocking out most of the sky. Little vegetation grows in the narrows because floods regularly scour the riverbed. At mile 7.2, Buckskin Canyon enters from the right through a narrow slot. You also cross the state line back into Arizona at this point, a fact that seems pretty irrelevant deep within the canyons.

Tip: In a pinch, you can hike about 0.25 mile up Buckskin Canyon to a broad alluvial terrace, which is the only spot in the Narrows section where you could escape rising water.

The Paria River is sometimes dry from the trailhead to Buckskin Canyon, but it usually flows downstream of this point. Buckskin Canyon offers an optional side hike.

Another 3 miles of hiking leads out of the narrows, which ends gradually as the canyon grows steadily deeper and wider. The first sign that the character of the canyon is changing is the appearance of Fremont cottonwood trees on alluvial terraces on the insides of bends. Watch for the first springs along the canyon walls. Although it still should be treated, the spring water is cleaner and certainly tastes better than the Paria River water. These terraces offer reasonable campsites safely above possible flood waters.

As you continue downstream, the canyon increases in depth and width. More sunlight finds its way to the bottom of the canyon, allowing cottonwoods and other vegetation to flourish. Watch for several rincons perched above the riverbed. Rincons are old canyon meanders that have been cut off from the main canyon. In a rincon, the now-abandoned river channel curves around a central sandstone butte. A particularly accessible rincon is located just above Judd Hollow, at mile 17.7. Judd Hollow marks a place where early ranchers attempted to pump water from the Paria River to the dry plateau above, in order to water their cattle. A few artifacts remain from this failed endeavor.

At mile 20 Wrather Canyon, a major side canyon, enters from the right. The canyon itself is a huge opening in the right wall of Paria Canyon, but the actual bed of the canyon enters the Paria through a narrow slot. Wrather Canyon offers an optional side hike.

After Wrather Canyon, Paria Canyon continues to grows wider, and the constant meanders decrease as the Paria River wanders generally east.

Tip: You can expect to find the last spring at around mile 25, so you may want to pick up water for camp farther down the canyon.

At mile 28, the canyon widens significantly, and the Paria River enters an open valley that leads down to Lees Ferry and the Colorado River.

Tip: You'll find little shade in this section. In hot weather, it's a good idea to camp near Water Pockets Canyon, at mile 28.5, and get an early start in order to walk the lower canyon in the cool of morning.

Below Water Pockets Canyon, an unmaintained trail offers an alternate route. As you near Lees Ferry you'll pass the ruins of the historic Lonely Dell Ranch, operated by John D. Lee and his wife. She supposedly exclaimed, "Oh, what a lonely dell!" when she first set eyes on her new home. Lee operated a ferry across the Colorado River just upstream from the mouth of the Paria River until the late 1920's, when Navajo Bridge replaced it. Even today, Colorado River crossings are far apart—the next bridged crossings upstream are at Page, 17 miles upstream, and Narrow Canyon, 200 miles above Lees Ferry. Downstream, the next bridged crossing is at Hoover Dam, 300 miles away.

At mile 34, the obscure Dominguez Pass Trail climbs 2 miles and 1600 feet to the east rim of the Canyon. Although it offers fine views of lower Paria Canyon, this trail is not often hiked because most backpackers have their sights set on Lees Ferry and a shower by this time.

POSSIBLE ITINERARY

	Camp	Miles	Elevation Gain
Day 1	End of Narrows	10.0	0
Day 2	Wrather Arch	10.1	0
Day 3	Water Pockets Canyon	8.3	0
Day 4	Out	8.6	0

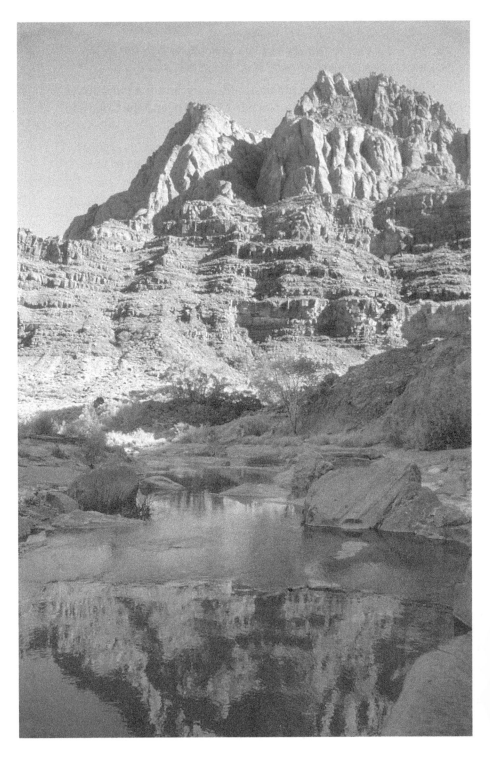

Paria River, Paria Canyon

⛰ Canyon Formation

Deep, narrow canyons form on the Colorado Plateau for several reasons. First, the entire plateau has been raised high above sea level, creating a huge amount of erosive power from the precipitation that falls on it. Second, an energetic Colorado River system is fed by copious snowfall in the Rocky Mountains, creating a master canyon and drainage to the sea. Third, the soft sandstone is eroded more rapidly by stream action than from local rainfall, so the canyon deepens quickly but widens slowly.

BUCKSKIN CANYON OPTIONAL SIDE HIKE Buckskin Canyon is 16 miles long, its width varies from 3 to 15 feet, and is up to 500 feet deep. A recommended side hike from Paria takes you 3 miles up the canyon. You'll encounter a boulder jam about 2 miles above the confluence with the Paria River. Steps cut into the rock form a bypass and you will need a rope to haul packs. A full-length hike of Buckskin Canyon is a more serious undertaking than the Paria, because you'll probably have to swim deep, cold pools.

WRATHER CANYON OPTIONAL SIDE HIKE A side hike of 0.6 mile and 200 feet elevation gain up Wrather Canyon takes you to a view of Wrather Arch, a spectacular hole through a fin projecting from the north wall of the canyon. Arches of this type are created when weathering erodes both sides of a fin, eventually cutting through at the base and forming an arch. Arches, in contrast to natural bridges, do not span stream courses.

UNMAINTAINED TRAIL ALTERNATE ROUTE Below Water Pockets Canyon, an unmaintained trail stays on the alluvial banks above the Paria River. You can either follow this trail or continue along the Paria River bed.

Tip: This trail can speed up the descent of the final stretch considerably, as it avoids several rocky sections of the riverbed.

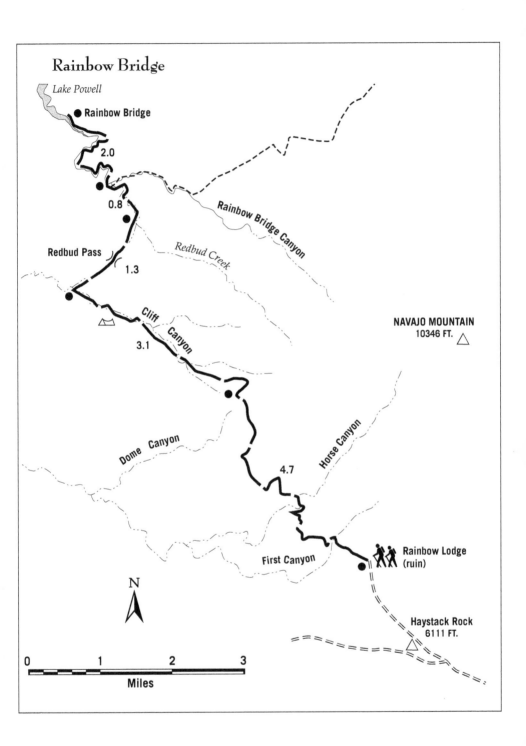

Rainbow Bridge

Lake Powell

● Rainbow Bridge

2.0

0.8

Redbud Pass

Redbud Creek

Rainbow Bridge Canyon

1.3

Cliff Canyon

3.1

NAVAJO MOUNTAIN
10346 FT. △

Dome Canyon

Horse Canyon

4.7

First Canyon

Rainbow Lodge
(ruin)

N

Haystack Rock
6111 FT.

0   1   2   3
Miles

2 Rainbow Bridge

RATINGS (1–10)			MILES	ELEVATION GAIN	DAYS	SHUTTLE MILEAGE
Scenery	Solitude	Difficulty	23.9	4740	3	0
9	8	7				

MAPS Rainbow Bridge, Chaiyahi Flat U.S.G.S.

SEASON March–November.

BEST April, October.

WATER Seasonal in Cliff Canyon, permanent in Bridge Canyon and Lake Powell.

PERMITS Required.

RULES None.

CONTACT Navajo Nation, Recreational Resources Department, Box 308, Window Rock, Arizona 86515; (928) 871-6647, or (928) 871-4941. Rainbow Bridge itself lies in Rainbow Bridge National Monument, which is administered by Glen Canyon National Recreation Area.

HIGHLIGHTS Rainbow Bridge is the world's largest natural bridge, and one of the most graceful—a frozen rainbow of stone. Although most people now reach the bridge by boat on Lake Powell, the hike around Navajo Mountain is scenic enough in its own right—the bridge is frosting on the cake.

PROBLEMS The Rainbow Bridge Trail, though originally constructed for pack stock, is no longer maintained. Until you reach the bridge and the lake, you are in a very remote corner of the Navajo Reservation. All but experienced desert hikers should avoid this route from mid May through mid September, because of temperatures that reach 100°F. Lake Powell is the only dependable water source during the summer months.

HOW TO GET THERE From Tuba City on U.S. 160, drive 40 miles northeast, and turn left on Arizona 98. Drive 13 miles, and turn right on Navajo 16. This road is paved for about 15 miles, to Inscription House Trading Post, and then becomes a graded, sandy road. Turn left 29 miles from Arizona 98, onto the Rainbow Lodge road, which is usually unsigned. Drive 5 miles, and look for a dome-shaped rock formation, Haystack Rock, ahead. Take the road that goes to the right of Haystack Rock. Unless you have a high-clearance four-wheel-drive vehicle, park at the fork at Haystock Rock. The trailhead lies 1.8 miles up the road, at the west side of the ruins of the old Rainbow Lodge, on the southwest slopes of dome-shaped Navajo Mountain.

Warning: There have been vehicle break-ins at this isolated trailhead. Do not leave valuables in your car.

DESCRIPTION The old horse trail starts from the ruins of Rainbow Lodge, a former departure point for guided pack trips to Rainbow Bridge. It contours for about 0.5 mile along the slope through the pygmy forest of pinyon pine and juniper trees and crosses appropriately named First Canyon. This is the first of several canyons you'll cross. After contouring around First Canyon, the trail heads northwest across another pinyon-juniper slope. Since the miniature forest is open, there are sweeping views of the canyon country to the south and west.

Tip: Although the trip can be done as an overnight hike, it is much more enjoyable as a 3-day trip. Because of the long drive to the trailhead, you won't have a full day of hiking on the first and last days. Also, a 3-day trip lets you camp in isolated, spectacular Cliff Canyon or Redbud Creek, instead of at Rainbow Bridge, which is crowded with boaters. Plan your trip to allow plenty of time at Rainbow Bridge. You won't regret it, and you'll have a chance to have the bridge to yourself during lulls in the boat and airplane traffic, especially early in the morning or late in the day.

After crossing Horse Canyon and a smaller, unnamed drainage, the trail turns to the north. Ahead, massive walls of salmon-hued Navajo sandstone mark the head of Dome Canyon. The trail contours above the head of this impressive canyon and then crosses a small, narrow ridge. Here it starts the steep descent into Cliff Canyon, plunging more than 1700 feet in 1.3 miles. Once the trail reaches the bottom of the canyon, watch for water in the bed. You may find a few pools

▲▲ Natural Bridges

Natural bridges, such as Rainbow Bridge, are created when a stream erodes both sides of a meander. Much of the erosion in these desert canyons takes place during brief but violent floods caused by summer thunderstorms. The floodwater, containing sand, gravel, and boulders, gnaws away at the outsides of bends. Where a canyon loops back on itself, such erosion tends to cut through the narrowing fin of rock separating the two sides of the bend. When it succeeds, the stream takes the new shortcut, rapidly turning it into the main channel. Occasionally the top of the fin remains intact, bridging the new streambed. The underside of the stone bridge continues to erode away, mainly from weathering of the rock surface, and the size of the opening increases. Eventually, of course, the structure is weakened to the point of collapse. Geologically speaking, natural bridges are very short-lived formations.

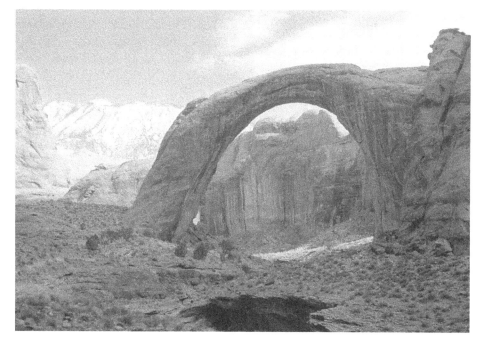

Rainbow Bridge

along this section. Pick up water for a dry camp, and then look for a campsite as you continue downstream. Plan to camp before you reach the turnoff to Redbud Pass.

▲▲ **Rainbow in Stone**

Rainbow Bridge spans 275 feet across the canyon and is 290 feet high, but the deep canyon dwarfs it. To put it in perspective, the dome of the U.S. Capitol would fit under the bridge. But numbers alone do not do Rainbow Bridge justice. Its graceful shape is indeed reminiscent of a rainbow. The Navajo, and several other Southwestern tribes, regard the bridge and its surroundings as an especially sacred site, and the name comes from a Navajo legend that tells of a rainbow frozen forever in stone. Please visit the bridge respectfully.

At 7.9 miles, the trail turns abruptly right (northeast) and climbs up a narrow slot canyon to Redbud Pass, drops into Redbud Creek, and then turns left, downstream. You'll find more campsites along Redbud Creek and seasonal water in the creek and in Rainbow Bridge Canyon. At 10.1 miles the trail enters Rainbow Bridge Canyon and meets the little-traveled north side trail from Navajo Mountain Trading Post. This trail offers an alternate route to Rainbow Bridge from a different trailhead.

It is less than two miles to Rainbow Bridge, but the intricate twists and turns of the canyon hide the massive stone arch until you reach the remains of an old camp at 11.7 miles. From the old camp, it's a short walk to the bridge itself. Beyond the bridge, the wellbeaten trail continues to the boat dock on the lake. You'll find no facilities at this dock, and camping is not permitted near the bridge.

POSSIBLE ITINERARY

	Camp	Miles	Elevation Gain
Day 1	Cliff Canyon	7.9	900
Day 2	Cliff Canyon	8.1	740
Day 3	Out	7.9	3100

NORTH SIDE TRAIL ALTERNATE ROUTE Another trail to Rainbow Bridge starts north of the old Navajo Mountain Trading Post, which is reached by continuing straight at the road junction 29 miles north

▲▲ Laccolithic Mountains

As you look east through Rainbow Bridge, Navajo Mountain is framed majestically under its span. The 10,346-foot, dome-shaped mountain is one of the sacred mountains that the Navajo believe form the four pillars supporting the sky. It formed when volcanic magma pushed upward into the horizontal sedimentary rocks to create the plateau. The liquid rock lifted the rocks above into a huge blister, but failed to reach the surface to create a volcano. As the dome of rock eroded, the solidified magma at its core was revealed. Today the rounded summit of Navajo Mountain consists of the exposed, intruded core, while the flanks of the mountain are draped with upturned layers of Navajo sandstone. These tilted have eroded into towering fins and buttresses, visible from the trail just before the descent into Cliff Canyon.

of Arizona 98. Drive about 13 miles, past Rainbow City, to the end of the road at the trailhead. The trail, which follows the route used by the Cummings–Douglas party in 1909, circles the north side of the mountain and joins the Rainbow Lodge Trail after 11.1 miles. It's another 1.8 miles down Rainbow Bridge Canyon to the bridge. This is a remote, unmaintained trail that traverses spectacular canyon country.

🪜 Exploration of Rainbow Bridge

Navajo Bridge was first publicized by the Cummings–Douglass party in 1909 after a long, difficult journey from Oljeto Trading Post, 50 miles to the east. The group brought back such glowing reports of the sandstone bridge that President Taft used the Antiquities Act to create Rainbow Bridge National Monument the following year. A few tourists reached the remote bridge during the next few decades, but to do so they had to make an arduous pack trip of many days from Oljeto. Later, the trail was built, shortening the journey considerably. In the 1950s Rainbow Bridge became a popular side hike for river runners traversing the depths of Glen Canyon on the Colorado River. It was still a 7-mile hike from the Colorado River, up Forbidding and Rainbow Bridge Canyons. Mass tourism at Rainbow Bridge began with the filling of Lake Powell in the 1960s, which marked the end of the bridge's isolation. Now Rainbow Bridge is a major destination for private boaters, tour boats, and aircraft.

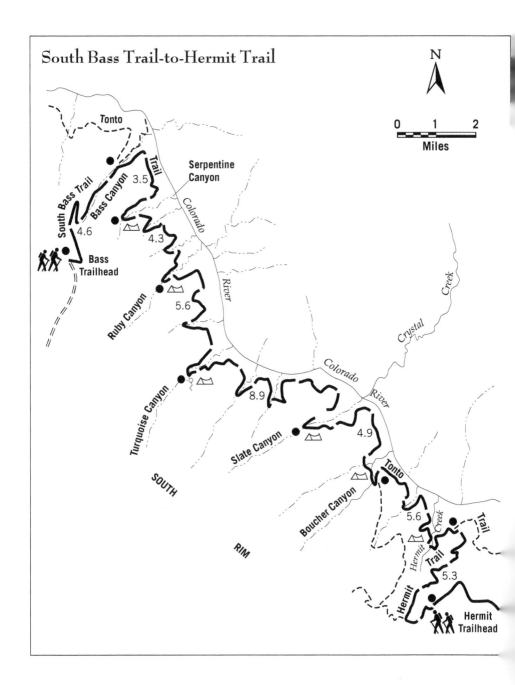

South Bass Trail-to-Hermit Trail

N

0 1 2
Miles

Tonto

South Bass Trail

Bass Canyon

Trail

3.5

Serpentine Canyon

Colorado

4.6

4.3

Bass Trailhead

Ruby Canyon

5.6

River

Turquoise Canyon

8.9

Colorado

River

Slate Canyon

4.9

Crystal Creek

SOUTH

Tonto

Boucher Canyon

5.6

Crystal Creek

RIM

Hermit Trail

Trail

5.3

Hermit Trail

Hermit Trailhead

3   South Bass Trail to Hermit Trail

RATINGS (1–10)			MILES	ELEVATION GAIN	DAYS	SHUTTLE MILEAGE
Scenery	Solitude	Difficulty	42.7	5970	5	36.8
10	7	6				

MAPS Havasupai Point, Shiva Temple, Grand Canyon, Piute Point U.S.G.S.

SEASON Mid September–May.

BEST October–November, March–April.

WATER Serpentine Canyon, Turquoise Canyon, Slate Creek, Boucher Creek, and Hermit Creek.

PERMITS Required for camping within Grand Canyon National Park.

RULES Campfires are not allowed in the national park backcountry. Pets are not allowed on trails or in the backcountry in the national park.

CONTACT Grand Canyon National Park, P.O. Box 129, Grand Canyon, Arizona 86023, (928) 638-7888, www.nps.gov/grca.

HIGHLIGHTS The Tonto Trail winds for over 70 miles along the Tonto Plateau through the eastern Grand Canyon. This hike covers the remote western half of this scenic trail. Starting from the South Bass Trail, the hike passes near the Grand Scenic Divide, where Grand Canyon geology changes dramatically. West of the Grand Scenic Divide, a red sandstone plateau called the Esplanade forms a major terrace about 1700 feet below the canyon rim. The Esplanade abruptly ends at the Grand Scenic Divide, and the Tonto Plateau takes over as the Grand Canyon's major mid-canyon terrace. This bench is about 3500 feet below the rim and reflects the gray-green color of its underlying shale rocks. Several side canyons allow side trips to the Colorado River and some of its major rapids, as well as exploration upstream.

PROBLEMS None of the trails are maintained and you will encounter trail damage and washouts. Your rate of progress will be slower than you expect. Water sources are far apart, and each hiker should have sufficient containers to carry water for an overnight dry camp.

> *Warning:* Map miles do not accurately reflect hiking distances in the Grand Canyon because of the rough terrain. This hike is dangerous during the summer. Do not attempt it from May through mid-September, when temperatures commonly exceed 100°F.

HOW TO GET THERE To reach the end trailhead from Grand Canyon Village on the South Rim, drive to the end of the West Rim Drive, and park at the Hermit Trailhead. During the summer season the West Rim Drive is closed to private vehicles. A free shuttle service is provided from Grand Canyon Village, so you will need to leave a vehicle there. The Bright Angel Trailhead at the west end of the village is a logical place to leave your vehicle because there is a shuttle bus stop there. To reach the starting trailhead, drive the Rowe Well Road west from the Bright Angel Trailhead. The road soon becomes graded dirt. Turn right 4.9 miles from the village. Drive 18.1 miles, and then turn right on the Pasture Wash Road. This road is not maintained and may be impassable during and after a wet winter because of deep mud. Continue 7.0 miles to the end of the road at the South Bass Trailhead.

DESCRIPTION The South Bass Trail descends to the east through open pinyon pine and juniper forest and switchbacks down to cross the head of Garnet Canyon. Eroded, short switchbacks take you through the Coconino sandstone.

Eventually the trail comes out onto the Esplanade, a broad terrace formed in the soft, red Hermit shale. The South Bass Trail can't descend the head of Bass Canyon because of the Esplanade sandstone cliff. Instead, it heads north along the west rim of the canyon for nearly a mile before finding such a fault break and descending. Once below the Esplanade sandstone, the trail rounds a point and doubles back toward the head of the canyon, exploiting breaks in the Supai sandstone layers as it finds them. It descends the Redwall limestone down to the bed of the canyon. Routes through the Redwall limestone are scarce because of the highly resistant nature of the limestone, and its constant thickness of more than 500 feet throughout the Grand Canyon. Only about 200 known routes have been discovered through the hundreds of miles of Redwall cliff exposed in the canyon. William Bass built his trail through one of these breaks, following an old Native American route.

▲▲▲ Rock Faults

Most of the trails and routes within the Grand Canyon take advantage of faults to descend through cliff-forming layers of rock such as the Esplanade sandstone. Faults are commonly formed when rock layers are pushed up or down and the rock fractures to allow the movement. The shattered rock erodes into ravines and slopes, creating routes through otherwise vertical cliffs.

Below the Redwall limestone gorge, Bass Canyon gradually opens up as the trail descends into the green and purple Bright Angel shale. Here, the trail stays mostly east of the bed. When the trail meets the brown, coarse Tapeats sandstone, it crosses the Tonto Trail. Turn right (east) on the Tonto Trail.

The South Bass Trail continues to the Colorado River, and is a worthwhile side trip. Of course, you can also go to the Colorado River for water.

Tip: You may find seasonal water at Bass Tanks, where the 7.5 minute topographic map shows a spring, about 0.7 mile north on the South Bass Trail.

Heading east on the Tonto Trail, you'll quickly find that the Tonto Plateau is not as level as it appears from the South Rim. In fact, it is remarkably rough. The trail dips into shallow ravines and winds around low ridges. The Tonto Trail also frequently climbs or descends to avoid obstacles. As compensation, the route alternates between spectacular points overlooking the Granite Gorge and the Colorado River, and the towering walls of side canyons. The trail eventually rounds the northeast end of the Grand Scenic Divide and heads southwest into Serpentine Canyon, the first of many named and unnamed side canyons. Serpentine Canyon usually has water where the Tonto Trail crosses it, and if not, it's an easy walk down the bed to the Colorado River. Serpentine Canyon, 8.4 miles from the South Bass Trailhead, makes a good first night's camping spot for small groups.

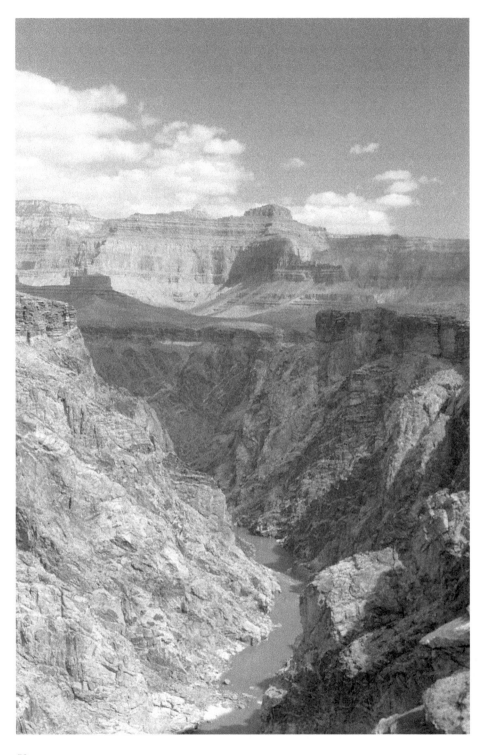

Granite Gorge from Tonto Trail

▲▲ Cliff and Terrace

In the canyon, the horizontal, sedimentary rock layers erode according to their hardness. Hard rocks such as limestone and sandstone form cliffs, while soft rocks such as shale and siltstone form slopes. Since these types of rocks tend to alternate in the cross section, the Grand Canyon has a staircase appearance of alternating cliffs and slopes. Terraces form where the soft layers are especially thick, so that the cliffs above retreat back and expose large, relatively level expanses of the lower cliff-forming layer. In the case of the Esplanade terrace along the upper South Bass Trail eastward, the surface of the terrace is formed on the upper sandstone member of the Supai formation (sometimes called the Esplanade sandstone), which tends to form a cliff about 200 feet high. In the central Grand Canyon, from the South Bass Trail westward, the Hermit shale thickens and causes the overlying Coconino sandstone to retreat back from the Esplanade Rim. Such terraces are vital for foot travel through the canyon. West of this point, the Esplanade forms the major route of travel. To the east, the Esplanade fades away because the Hermit shale is thinner. At the same time, the Bright Angel shale becomes thicker, forming a new terrace, the Tonto Plateau, on top of the resistant Tapeats sandstone. As you hike along the ridge at the head of Bass Canyon, you can look out at the Esplanade to the west, and down Bass Canyon at the Tonto Plateau to the north.

As the Tonto Trail continues southeast, it winds around three unnamed side canyons before reaching Ruby Canyon. Although you've hiked 4.6 miles on the Tonto Trail, you've come only 1.8 miles in a straight line from Serpentine Canyon. You may find seasonal water in Ruby Canyon, and it offers small camp sites. After the Tonto Trail rounds the point east of Ruby Canyon, it swings into and heads two more unnamed canyons before heading into Turquoise Canyon, 9.9 miles from Serpentine Canyon. You will probably find seasonal water in Turquoise Canyon, which has good campsites. Beyond Turquoise Canyon, the Tonto Trail continues east, following the general trend of the Grand Canyon itself. The trail winds nearly four miles rounding Sapphire and Agate Canyons. North of Agate, the Tonto Trail comes to the very edge of the Tonto Plateau and offers fine views of the Colorado River entrenched deep in Granite Gorge.

The trail works its way across gullies emanating from the base of Geikie Peak, and then rounds Scylla Butte to head into Slate Creek.

You'll find plentiful campsites at this popular spot, and there is almost always water below the point where the trail crosses the bed. A side hike down Slate Creek to the Colorado River is an option here.

▲▲ Granite Gorge

As you hike the portions of the Tonto Trail along the rim of Granite Gorge, you can clearly see that the brownish Tapeats sandstone forms a persistent cliff about 200 feet high along the rim of Granite Gorge. The gorge itself is cut into highly resistant, grayish rocks known as the Vishnu schist. These somber, twisted rocks are the metamorphosed roots of ancient mountains, and are among the oldest rocks on earth.

After leaving Slate Creek, the Tonto Trail rounds Marsh Butte, another summit formed at the end of a massive ridge of Redwall limestone, and heads into Topaz Canyon. It descends into Topaz Canyon to cross at the confluence with Boucher Creek. The Tonto Trail then follows Boucher Creek upstream to Boucher Camp. Boucher Camp is the site of Louis Boucher's old camp and mine. Boucher was a reclusive prospector who built two trails into this region of the Grand Canyon. Remains of his stone cabin are still visible. Boucher Creek offers plenty of campsites. You'll normally find flowing water near the trail crossing, or just up or downstream. An optional side hike down Boucher Creek to the Colorado River is possible here as well.

The Tonto Trail leaves Boucher Camp via an unnamed side canyon to the south. After it climbs back above the Tapeats, the Boucher Trail forks to the right. Our route continues north on the Tonto Trail and east into Travertine Canyon. After leaving this rough, dry canyon, the trail leads around a point and into Hermit Canyon, via a detour, and crosses a small, unnamed canyon.

Hermit Creek is one of the few permanent streams on the south side of the Colorado River, and since it is reached by a relatively good trail, it's a popular spot. The Park Service restricts camping to two places, one just below the point where the Tonto Trail crosses the creek, and another at the Colorado River at the mouth of Hermit Canyon. The delightful stream, which comes from springs at the base of the Redwall limestone, makes Hermit Canyon a treat. An optional side hike goes down Hermit Creek to the Colorado River.

~~~ Rock Made by Springs

Travertine Canyon is named for the massive formations of travertine rock found there. Travertine is a limestone-like rock formed by mineral-laden streams as the water evaporates in the desert air. Such springs and creeks actively create travertine elsewhere in the Grand Canyon, so the presence of travertine here proves that water once flowed freely in Travertine Canyon and probably year round.

After the Tonto Trail climbs out on the east side of Hermit Canyon, you'll pass the remains of Hermit Camp. In the early years of the twentieth century, this tent camp was the major tourist destination within the canyon. The Hermit Trail was improved to allow access, and an aerial tram brought supplies down from Pima Point on the South Rim. When the trans-canyon Kaibab Trail was completed in the late 1920s, Phantom Ranch was established at the mouth of Bright Angel Creek, and Hermit Camp was abandoned.

Northeast of the old camp, as you approach a saddle on the Tonto Trail, turn right onto the Hermit Trail. The trail switchbacks up the increasingly steep slope of Bright Angel shale, and then climbs into a ravine at the base of the Redwall limestone. The trail climbs this fault ravine through the Redwall via a series of short switchbacks known as the Cathedral Stairs, and then heads around Breezy Point and starts ascending the Supai formation. Long traverses are interrupted by short climbs as the trail takes advantage of breaks in the Supai cliffs. Some maps still show Four Mile Spring, but it has been dry for many years. The trail goes all the way past Santa Maria Spring before finding a way through the Esplanade sandstone at the top of the Supai formation. Don't count on Santa Maria Spring for water, as it is often dry.

▲▲ Sand Dunes Frozen in Time

Throughout most of the canyon, the Coconino sandstone forms a buff-colored cliff about 350 feet high, forming a distinct cliff band and serious obstacle about 500 feet below the rim. Look closely at the sandstone as you descend through it on the South Bass Trail or climb through it on the Hermit Trail, and you'll see that it is composed of many tilted layers. Observation with a microscope reveals that the individual sand grains are rough and pitted, which indicates that they were tumbled in the wind, rather than in water. This, along with the tilted cross-bedding, shows that the Coconino sandstone was deposited in a Sahara-like desert—a sea of ancient sand dunes.

After the trail climbs into Hermit Basin, it meets the Dripping Spring Trail coming in from the right, and then the Waldron Trail (also on the right) after it starts the ascent of the slope to the east. The ascent through the Coconino sandstone is marked by serious trail construction, where the trail was paved with slabs of rock placed edgewise. Fossil reptile tracks are visible on a slab at one point during the ascent of the Hermit Trail through the Coconino sandstone. The trail swings around to the north to find a break through the Toroweap formation, and then switchbacks up to Hermits Rest and the trailhead.

POSSIBLE ITINERARY

	Camp	Miles	Elevation Gain
Day 1	Serpentine Canyon	8.1	0
Day 2	Turquoise Canyon	9.9	1050
Day 3	Slate Creek	8.9	720
Day 4	Hermit Creek	9.4	450
Day 5	Out	6.4	3730

SLATE CREEK OPTIONAL SIDE HIKE It is possible to descend Slate Creek to the Colorado River. This side hike takes you to Crystal Rapid, one of the ten most difficult rapids in the Grand Canyon.

BOUCHER CREEK OPTIONAL SIDE HIKE From Boucher Camp, you can easily hike down Boucher Creek to the Colorado River. This easy cross-country hike takes you to Boucher Rapid, an easy one as Grand Canyon rapids go.

HERMIT CREEK OPTIONAL SIDE HIKE An informal trail follows Hermit Creek downstream to the Colorado River and Hermit Rapid. Hermit Rapid is noted more for its big waves than its technical difficulty.

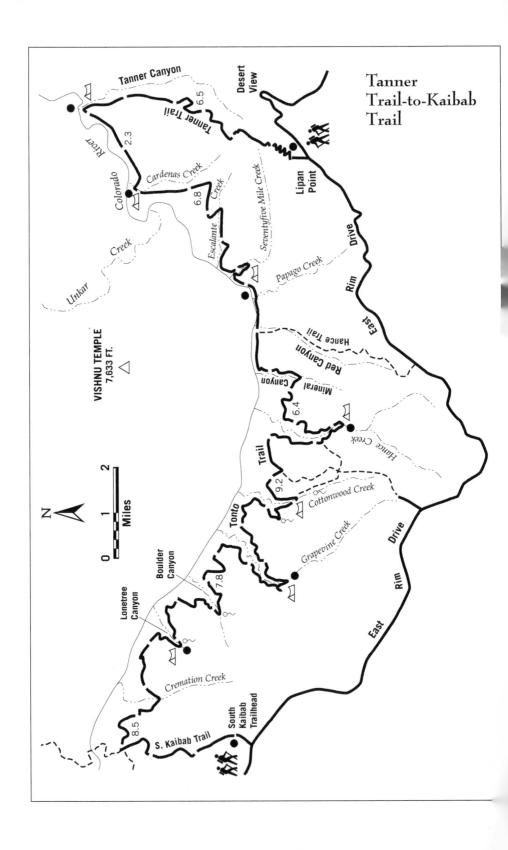

4 Tanner Trail to Kaibab Trail

RATINGS (1–10)			MILES	ELEVATION GAIN	DAYS	SHUTTLE MILEAGE
Scenery	Solitude	Difficulty	47.5	7580	6	25
10	6	7				

MAPS Desert View, Cape Royal, Grandview Point U.S.G.S.

SEASON Mid September–May.

BEST October–November, March–April.

WATER Colorado River, Hance Creek, Cottonwood Creek, Grapevine Creek, Boulder Canyon, and Lonetree Canyon.

PERMITS Required for camping within Grand Canyon National Park.

RULES Campfires are not allowed in the national park backcountry. Pets are not allowed on trails or in the backcountry.

CONTACT Grand Canyon National Park, P.O. Box 129, Grand Canyon, Arizona 86023, (928) 638-7888, www.nps.gov/grca.

HIGHLIGHTS This hike initially descends into the eastern section of the Grand Canyon, where the geology is strikingly different from the central Grand Canyon. Here, the soft rocks of the Precambrian Grand Canyon series are exposed. These colorful shales and sandstones have eroded into a relatively open space along the Colorado River, as compared to the deep Granite Gorge along the western section of this hike. The stretch of the Colorado River through Granite Gorge features some of the wildest rapids in the Grand Canyon. Optional side hikes take you to several of these long, rocky, and violent rapids.

PROBLEMS The South Kaibab Trail is the only maintained trail on this hike. The Tanner and Tonto Trails are unmaintained, and there is a section of cross-country hiking. Your rate of progress will be slower than you expect. Water sources are far apart, and each hiker should have sufficient containers to carry water for an overnight dry camp.

HOW TO GET THERE To reach the starting point at the Tanner Trailhead from Grand Canyon Village, drive south 0.7 mile past Mather Point, turn left onto the East Rim Drive and drive 23 miles to the Lipan Point turnoff and turn left. Park in the view point parking area. The South Kaibab Trailhead, the end of the hike, is reached by shuttle bus from Grand Canyon Village. Private cars are not allowed at the South Kaibab Trailhead, so you will have to leave your vehicle in the village.

Warning: Map miles do not accurately reflect hiking distances in the Grand Canyon because of the rough terrain. This hike is dangerous during the summer. Do not attempt it from May through mid September, when temperatures commonly exceed 100°F.

DESCRIPTION The Tanner Trail starts from the signed trailhead on the east side of the Lipan Point parking lot. The trail plunges down the head of Tanner Canyon in a series of short, steep switchbacks, quickly passing through the rim cliffs of Kaibab limestone. After about a mile the trail comes out on the narrow saddle between Seventyfive Mile Creek and Tanner Canyon. Follow the Tanner Trail around Escalante and Cardenas Buttes to the break through the Redwall limestone.

▲▲ Gravity Faults

Escalante and Cardenas Buttes have been studied for their gravity faults. As the buttes erode and are separated from the rim, their weight squeezes the softer rocks at their bases like toothpaste, causing the buttes to sink and tilt toward the Colorado River. This creates small faults, with a displacement of just a few feet.

Tip: There is no water along the Tanner Trail. Be sure to carry all you will need to reach the Colorado River at the end of the Tanner Trail, a distance of 6.5 miles.

The Tanner Trail goes nearly to the end of the Redwall point northeast of Cardenas Butte before finding the break in the 550-foot Redwall limestone cliff. It descends the Redwall via a series of switchbacks, and then turns north through scattered picturesque blocks of Tapeats sandstone. The final descent to the Colorado River stays mostly on the east side of the ridge, and then drops into the bed of Tanner Canyon for the last few yards to the Colorado River. Campsites are easy to find in the relatively open space along the Colorado River.

To continue the hike, follow the informal but distinct trail downriver (southwest) from the foot of the Tanner Trail. Although never an official, constructed trail, in recent years enough hikers have traveled from Tanner Canyon to Red Canyon to create a good trail. For a short distance the Colorado River races by almost underfoot, but then the trail moves back to follow the easiest route, well above the brushy riverbank. Hike 2.3 miles to the mouth of Cardenas Creek. You'll find plenty of campsites here also, and the Colorado River is close at hand.

Hike up Cardenas Creek through a short narrows, and then continue upstream.

Tip: *Carry plenty of water, because you will be away from the Colorado River for most of the day and there is no water along the route.*

Multiple trails confuse this area, but just work your way west onto the ridge crest overlooking Unkar Rapid, and then follow the trail south up the ridge. After about a mile of ridge-top walking, the trail turns onto the west slope of the ridge, then swings west around the head of a nameless canyon. It continues west for another mile, below an impressive palisade of Tapeats sandstone, before contouring around the end of the ridge.

Tanner Trail and the Horse Thieves

Like most Grand Canyon trails, the Tanner Trail was built by prospectors to reach mineral deposits in the depths of the canyon. Unlike most, the Tanner Trail never became a major tourist trail. One early party had their horses stolen from the rim, which implies that horse thieves were using the Tanner Trail as part of a trans-canyon route to secretly move stolen horses. The story had it that thieves would steal horses in New Mexico, then take them down the Tanner Trail, across the Colorado River, and out to the north rim via the Nankoweap Trail, and on to Utah where they would sell the horses. The thieves used this torturous Grand Canyon route to avoid the normal crossings of the Colorado River upstream at Lees Ferry and Hite Ferry, where it would be impossible to cross unobserved.

The trail drops rapidly into Escalante Creek and turns downstream, heading west toward the Colorado River. After another mile, the trail suddenly veers out of the bed of Escalante Creek to the left to avoid a dry fall. It drops into a tributary and returns to Escalante Creek below the obstacle, only to encounter another dry fall near the Colorado River. The trail avoids the dry fall on the left and descends to the Colorado River.

Continue downstream along the Colorado River, where a rising cliff of Shinumo quartzite, part of the Grand Canyon series, falls directly into the Colorado River and forces the trail to follow a ramp rising above the water. Just 0.5 mile downstream from Escalante Creek, you'll encounter the deep, narrow gorge of lower Seventyfive Mile Creek where it meets the Colorado River. The trail turns upstream along the rim of this little canyon, and continues 0.5 mile until the gorge ends and you can make your way into the dry bed of Seventyfive Mile Creek. Follow the bed 0.5 mile downstream through the narrows to the Colorado River. Now, turn left and follow the Colorado River downstream once again. You'll find plenty of campsites from here to Papago Creek.

At Papago Creek, 0.7 mile downstream, cliffs falling directly into the Colorado River once again block the Colorado River level route. To bypass this obstacle, climb up ledges just right (west) of

≋ Stream Capture

The unnamed saddle at the head of Seventyfive Mile Canyon not only offers a fine view, it is also the site of a soon-to-occur geologic event: soon in geologic time, that is. The head of Seventyfive Mile Creek plunges rapidly west of the saddle. Side canyons become deeper primarily by erosion at the head of the canyon, where steep gradients cause rapid downcutting by storm runoff. The canyon gnaws into the cliffs at its head much like a child digging into a sandhill. In contrast, the bed along the middle and lower portions of a canyon has a gentler gradient, causing downcutting to proceed at a slower rate. To the east, the middle section of Tanner Canyon is downcutting its bed at a slower rate than the head of Seventyfive Mile Creek to the west of the saddle. As Seventyfive Mile Creek deepens, it pushes eastward. When it reaches the bed of Tanner Canyon, it will capture the drainage. Upper Tanner Canyon will then become the new head of Seventyfive Mile Creek.

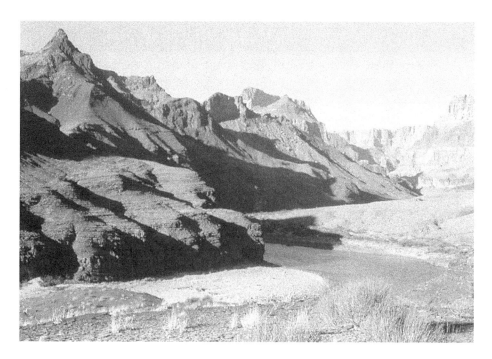

Foot of the Tanner Trail at the Colorado River

Papago Creek until you are about 200 feet above the Colorado River. Although there often isn't a trail on the bare rock, rock cairns usually mark the route. Once high enough, the route traverses west to a ravine that descends through the cliffs and leads you back to the Colorado River. It's now an easy 0.6 mile along the riverside trail to the mouth of Red Canyon.

At Red Canyon, you meet the junction of the Hance Trail and the Tonto Trail. It's possible to camp here, but the area is sandy and there's little protection from wind. Continue the hike west on the Tonto Trail, which follows a rising ramp above the Colorado River. This gives you good views of long, rocky Hance Rapid, one of the hardest in the canyon, especially at low water. As you climb, you also get glimpses of the beginnings of Granite Gorge. Travel along the Colorado River's edge is impossible in Granite Gorge, so the Tonto Trail follows the slope of the last of the Grand Canyon series as they are pinched out against the rising schist, and climbs west into Mineral Canyon. The trail continues south 1.0 mile up the east side of Mineral Canyon before crossing to the west and climbing to the top of the Tapeats sandstone and the Tonto Plateau. With only brief exceptions, the Tonto Trail stays on top of the Tapeats sandstone from here westward. The Tonto Trail soon reaches the east rim of Hance Canyon, which forms an obstacle requiring a 4.1-mile detour in order to progress 0.4 mile westward. Such is travel along the Tonto!

Tip: Where the trail crosses Hance Creek, you can usually find water by walking downstream toward the Tapeats narrows.

The Temple of Set, a huge overhang below the narrows, provides shelter on a stormy day. You'll find plenty of campsites both above and below the narrows.

▲▲▲ Grand Canyon Series of Rocks

The open feel of the eastern Grand Canyon is because the lowest layers of rock are mostly soft, slope-forming shales. These rocks are part of the Grand Canyon series, and one way to distinguish them from the overlying younger rocks is by their tilt. The sedimentary rocks that now make up the Grand Canyon series were laid down horizontally, like all such rocks, and then later tilted by ancient mountain building movements. The horizontal, purplish-brown Tapeats sandstone forms an abrupt cap on top of the Grand Canyon series.

Continue the hike on the Tonto Trail north along the west rim of Hance Canyon, then west past the two prongs of Horseshoe Mesa. The Tonto Trail continues across the main arm of Cottonwood Creek to a tributary of Cottonwood Creek, which has a few small campsites and usually water.

Continue west on the Tonto Trail around the Redwall spur between Cottonwood and Grapevine Canyons. Then hike southwest along the east rim of Grapevine Canyon to reach the the bed of Grapevine Canyon and several campsites. Grapevine Canyon is a logical overnight stop. You can usually find water in Grapevine Canyon, especially downstream of the Tonto Trail crossing.

Tip: If the weather has been dry, carry enough water for one night's dry camp when you leave Grapevine Canyon. In warm weather or drought periods, there may be no water between Grapevine and your exit on the South Kaibab Trail.

At 7533 feet, pyramid-shaped Vishnu Temple towers well above the south rim and dominates the views to the north along this section of the Tonto Trail. Often called the Matterhorn of the Grand Canyon, its distinctive spire is visible throughout the eastern canyon. As in much of the West, early visitors named most of the summits in the canyon. Because of the inaccessibility of the Grand Canyon region, many of the first explorers were scientists such as geologists John Wesley Powell and Clarence Dutton. Dutton in particular drew on mythology for place names, which explains Vishnu Temple and its satellites Krishna Shrine and Rama Shrine. Powell is responsible for many other names such as Bright Angel Creek.

Continue the hike on the Tonto Trail west of Grapevine Canyon. Actually, the trail heads northeast along the west rim of Grapevine Canyon before rounding the Redwall spur to the west. This section of the Tonto Trail skirts the very brink of Granite Gorge above Grapevine Rapid and provides views of the Colorado River. After heading a nameless canyon, the Tonto Trail heads southwest into Boulder Canyon. If the seasonal unnamed spring in Boulder Canyon has water, top off your containers. Access to the Colorado River for water is impossible between Grapevine Canyon and the South Kaibab Trail.

After leaving Boulder Canyon, the Tonto Trail heads north around another nameless canyon before turning west into Lonetree Canyon. Lonetree Canyon has a seasonal unnamed spring, and this is a logical place to camp before ascending the South Kaibab Trail on your last day.

West of Lonetree Canyon, the Tonto Trail rounds several major Redwall spurs radiating from Pattie Butte before reaching Cremation Creek. Cremation Creek offers plenty of campsites but is normally dry. After crossing the three arms of Cremation Canyon, the Tonto Trail climbs gradually to cross the South Kaibab Trail, a maintained and heavily used trail. Turn left (south) on the South Kaibab Trail, and start the steady climb to the rim.

South of the Tonto Trail junction, the South Kaibab Trail gradually ascends the Bright Angel shale slopes. Watch for a small natural arch on the Redwall skyline to the west, before the trail reaches the base of the Redwall limestone. The South Kaibab Trail ascends the Redwall via a series of short switchbacks, and then heads south along the top

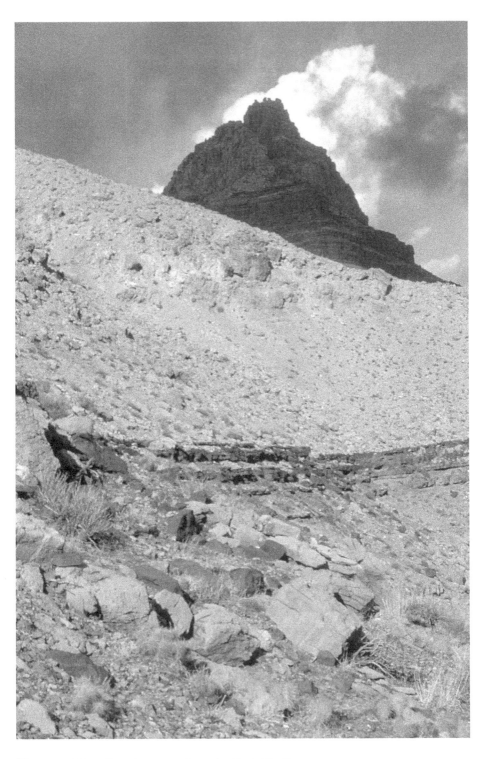

Vishnu Temple as seen from the Tonto Trail

Unlike most Grand Canyon trails, the Kaibab did not follow a prehistoric route or prospector's trail. When Grand Canyon became a National Park in 1916, the Bright Angel Trail was in private hands. Since it was the only trail from Grand Canyon Village to the Colorado River, the owners had a monopoly and charged a hefty fee to use the trail. The Park Service initially failed in their efforts to buy the Bright Angel Trail and built the South Kaibab Trail as an alternative. The South Kaibab Trail was engineered to follow a constant grade, and there are few level sections. After a few years, the Park Service succeeded in buying the Bright Angel, which is why there are now two maintained trails from the south rim to the Colorado River.

of the Redwall toward O'Neill Butte. It ascends around O'Neill on the east and climbs Cedar Ridge through the remainder of the red shale, limestone, and sandstone layers of the Supai formation. The South Kaibab Trail ascends through the Coconino sandstone below Yaki Point. A brief traverse across slopes in the Toroweap formation leads to the final switchbacks through the Kaibab limestone to the South Kaibab Trailhead. From the trailhead you can take the shuttle bus into Grand Canyon Village and your vehicle.

POSSIBLE ITINERARY

	Camp	Miles	Elevation Gain
Day 1	Cardenas Creek	8.8	0
Day 2	Papago Creek	6.8	1580
Day 3	Hance Creek	6.4	1530
Day 4	Grapevine Creek	9.2	330
Day 5	Lonetree Canyon	7.8	410
Day 6	Out	8.5	3730

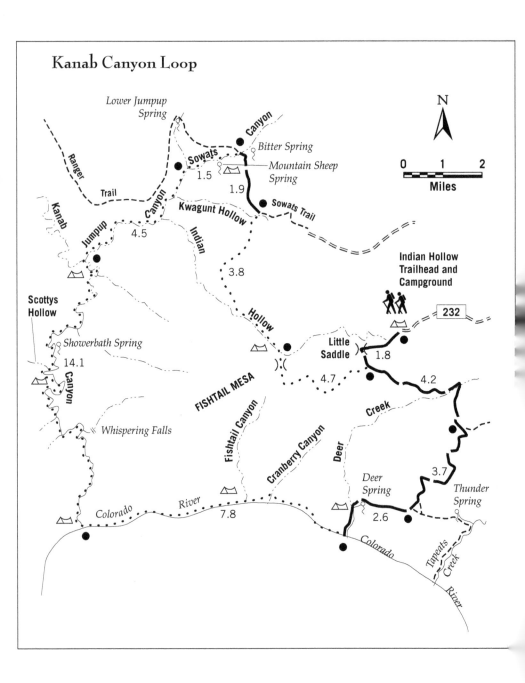

Kanab Canyon Loop

Lower Jumpup Spring

Sowats Canyon

Bitter Spring

Mountain Sheep Spring

1.5

1.9

Sowats Trail

Ranger

Trail

Kwagunt Hollow

Kanab

Jumpup Canyon

4.5

Indian

3.8

Hollow

Indian Hollow Trailhead and Campground

232

Little Saddle

1.8

4.7

4.2

Scottys Hollow

Showerbath Spring

14.1

Canyon

FISHTAIL MESA

Whispering Falls

Fishtail Canyon

Cranberry Canyon

Deer Creek

Deer Spring

3.7

Thunder Spring

Colorado

River

7.8

2.6

Colorado

Tapeats Creek

River

N

0 1 2

Miles

5   Kanab Canyon Loop

RATINGS (1–10)			MILES	ELEVATION GAIN	DAYS	SHUTTLE MILEAGE
Scenery	Solitude	Difficulty	52.2	5570	7	0
10	9	9				

MAPS Sowats Spring, Jumpup Point, Kanab Point, Fishtail, Tapeats Amphitheater U.S.G.S.

SEASON March–mid May, mid September–November.

BEST March–April, October.

WATER Kanab Creek, Colorado River, and Deer Creek, and seasonally in Indian Hollow and at Mountain Sheep Spring.

PERMITS Required for camping within Grand Canyon National Park.

RULES Campfires are not allowed in the national park backcountry. Pets are not allowed on trails or in the backcountry.

CONTACT Grand Canyon National Park, P.O. Box 129, Grand Canyon, Arizona 86023, (928) 638-7888, www.nps.gov/grca.

HIGHLIGHTS This excellent loop trip goes through remote sections of the Grand Canyon. Highlights include the deep Redwall limestone gorges of Jumpup and Kanab Canyons, an enjoyable cross-country hike along the Colorado River, and Deer Creek Falls. There's an optional side hike to Thunder River, which bursts suddenly out of a cave. Kanab Canyon features several side canyons with grottos and seasonal waterfalls, and one of the most unusual springs in the Grand Canyon.

PROBLEMS Much of this loop is strenuous cross-country hiking. All members of the party should be fit, and the leader should have experience hiking cross-country in the Grand Canyon. Those without such experience should choose one of the on-trail Grand Canyon hikes—Tanner Trail to Kaibab Trail, or South Bass Trail to Hermit

Trail. You must have the U.S.G.S. 7.5 minute topographic maps for critical route finding on this hike. Water sources are often far apart, and each hiker should have enough water containers to carry water for an overnight dry camp.

Warning: *This is a dangerous hike during the summer because of high temperatures, difficult terrain, and lack of water. Do not attempt this hike from May through mid September, when temperatures commonly exceed 100°F.*

Do not underestimate the difficulty of this hike. Your rate of progress may average one mile per hour, and can fall to half a mile per hour at times. Map miles do not accurately reflect hiking distances in the Grand Canyon because of the rough terrain.

Stay out of the Jumpup Canyon narrows if it is flowing, or if there is any chance of a thunderstorm in its watershed. Do not camp in areas subject to flooding. Distant storms can cause flash floods with little warning.

In addition, this hike may be impossible during heavy periods of runoff in Kanab Creek, which are common during the spring and may occur during late summer thunderstorms.

HOW TO GET THERE From Jacob Lake at the junction of U.S. 89A and Arizona 67, head south 0.4 mile on Arizona 67 and turn right (west) on Forest Road 461. Stay on this maintained dirt road 5.1 miles and bear right on Forest Road 462. Continue 3.3 miles; turn left on Forest Road 22, the Big Springs Road. (During the spring, when the forest roads from Jacob Lake may still be snowed in, you can reach this junction via Forest Road 22 from Fredonia on U.S. 89A.) Drive 11.9 miles south; turn right on Forest Road 425. Another 8.3 miles brings you Forest Road 232, where you'll turn right. This road is unmaintained but usually passable to most cars. Continue to the end of the road at the Indian Hollow Trailhead.

Tip: *The small Forest Service campground at the trailhead is a handy place to stay at the start or end of your trip.*

DESCRIPTION The Thunder River Trail wanders down the Indian Hollow drainage 0.2 mile, giving no hint of the massive canyon complex just a few hundred yards away. When the trail veers left and climbs to Little Saddle, the Grand Canyon is suddenly revealed. Those who have only seen the Grand Canyon from the popular south rim overlooks may wonder why this section of the Grand Canyon looks different. Here, a terrace is formed on the top of the reddish Supai formation. This broad terrace, called the Esplanade, is just 1500 feet below the north rim in this region.

Follow the Thunder River Trail down the slope to the Esplanade. When the trail turns east, leave the trail and hike cross-country to the west (the Indian Hollow Trail will be our return route). You'll quickly find that the Esplanade is not quite as level and easy as it appears from above. Side canyons, large and small, constantly cut the sandstone surface, and you are always heading one of these dry drainages or swinging around a point.

Tip: *Maintain a level contour as much as you can.*

Sometimes the Esplanade rewards you with easy walking along broad rock terraces that form a smooth, level path. All too often, it offers you a choice of several levels. Pick the wrong level, and you'll struggle across steep talus at the back of a small canyon, while you can clearly see that the one below you offered clear sailing. Picking the right level becomes easier with experience.

As you continue east, watch for a large boulder marking an old cowboy camp, which is near the 4811T elevation point shown on the U.S.G.S. topographic map. This huge rock offers a rare bit of shade on the sage-covered terrace, and judging from the old tin cans and other debris, it was a popular stopping point when cattle were grazed within the canyons.

After the old campsite, contour around the east fork of Fishtail Canyon and swing around the point between the east and west forks. Above, to the northwest, you can clearly see the saddle between the north rim and Fishtail Mesa. Climb toward this saddle as the terrain permits. The final ascent to the saddle leads up a rockslide through the buff Coconino sandstone. Here you may find switchbacks from an old trail. Descend the easy slope on the north side of the pass to Indian Hollow. Continue down Indian Hollow about a mile to the Esplanade. This is a good place to camp, and you are likely to find water pockets on the bare sandstone of the Esplanade, or along the drainage.

Tip: *If the weather has been dry, you may want to carry water from the trailhead.*

Hike north along the Esplanade, and head the nameless canyon between Kwagunt Hollow and Indian Hollow. After you cross Kwagunt Hollow, you should pick up the Sowats Trail. Follow this little used trail north, and then down into Sowats Canyon. Leave the trail and descend through the Supai formation into Sowats Canyon. You should find water along Sowats Canyon and at Mountain Sheep Spring.

Tip: *Another possible source, though it is out of the way, is Lower Jumpup Spring, upstream in Jumpup Canyon.*

Follow Sowats Canyon downstream to Jumpup Canyon and turn left (downstream) in Jumpup Canyon. When the bed is dry, as it normally is, the walking is easy.

Warning: *Do not continue if Jumpup Canyon is flooding. The narrows downstream will be impassable.*

Soon you'll enter the impressive Redwall limestone narrows. Jumpup Canyon enters Kanab Canyon at a confluence of towering red and gray cliffs. You'll find campsites on the alluvial terraces along Kanab Creek, but both Kanab and Jumpup Creeks may be dry.

Turn left and hike down Kanab Canyon. Permanent springs create a perennial stream in Kanab Creek just two miles downstream from the mouth of Jumpup Canyon. As you boulder-hop downstream, the flow quickly gathers strength. You can't miss Showerbath Spring, which pours from an overhanging mass of travertine rock on the left side of the creek. As its name implies, the spring makes a fine, cool shower on a warm day. The bottom of Kanab Canyon is fairly broad, and there's no difficulty finding campsites.

Continuing down Kanab Canyon, you'll encounter several long Muav limestone ledges exposed along the east side of the creek, a sign that you are nearing the Colorado River. These long ledges are a welcome respite from the constant boulder hopping. When you reach the Colorado River, you're faced with crossing the lagoon at the mouth of the creek in order to continue upriver. When the Colorado River is high, the lagoon may be too deep to wade. In this case, cross Kanab Creek above the lagoon to reach an informal trail on the east side.

Warning: *The Colorado River rises and falls several feet a day as water is released at Glen Canyon Dam in response to electrical power loads. Do not camp close to river level.*

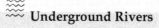

Underground Rivers

Large springs that burst suddenly out of Redwall limestone caves are found in several places in the Grand Canyon. Many other springs feed perennial streams which begin in the Redwall limestone. Kanab Creek is a prime example. Upper Kanab Creek flows intermittently, fed by snowmelt and storm runoff. When Kanab Creek encounters the base of the Redwall limestone, numerous springs appear. Why does so much water appear at the base of the Redwall limestone, when the plateaus to the north and south of the Grand Canyon are so dry? The surfaces of both plateaus are Kaibab limestone. Rain and snowmelt quickly soak into this porous rock, and continue down through the even more porous sandstone layers below. Water also seeps down through the Redwall limestone until it encounters the Bright Angel shale, which isn't nearly as porous. The groundwater tends to collect on top of the shale, in the Redwall limestone, forming an aquifer about 2000 feet below the surfaces of the plateaus. Where the Redwall limestone is exposed in the Grand Canyon, some of this water emerges as springs. Also, since water dissolves limestone, an extensive network of caverns has been carved out of the Redwall. At springs such as Deer Spring and Thunder Spring, parts of this cavern system have been exposed by erosion, and underground rivers have burst forth.

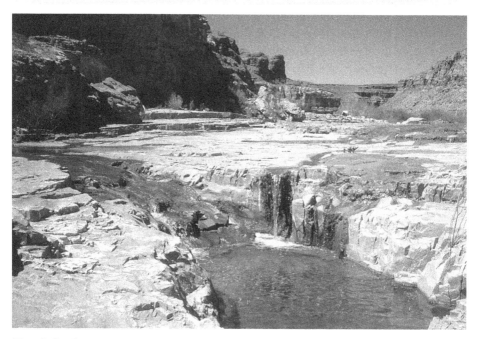

Kanab Creek

Hiking upriver involves more boulder hopping, though sandy striates offer a break as well as possible riverside campsites. The south-facing riverbank offers little shade, so if the weather is warm you may want to hike early in the morning or late in the day to avoid the worst of the heat.

At the mouth of Fishtail Canyon, you'll have to climb up a couple hundred feet onto a terrace to avoid cliffs that drop directly into the Colorado River.

Tip: *You'll be away from the Colorado River for a couple of miles, so pick up water at Fishtail Canyon.*

You may find traces of a trail to help you along this rough section. Shortly after reaching the terrace, you'll cross a nameless canyon referred to as "Cranberry Canyon" by most Grand Canyon hikers because the first party to find a way up this canyon did so on Thanksgiving Day. Another mile leads to rougher terrain as you cross several small canyons. Shortly after this, you can start descending to the Colorado River, and a final mile of cross-country hiking leads to the Deer Creek Trail and Deer Creek Falls. The falls are a famous destination for backpackers and river runners, for good reason. Deer Creek Falls shoots out of a narrow slot in the Tapeats sandstone and falls directly into a deep pool. If the Colorado River is high, the cascade may land in the Colorado River itself.

Continue the trip by following the Deer Creek Trail up switchbacks west of the falls. The trail contours into the narrow gorge above the falls. Follow the trail upstream along narrow ledges above the rushing creek.

Warning: *It's 12.3 miles and 4000' elevation gain from Deer Creek Valley to the Indian Hollow Trailhead. Carry plenty of water from Deer Creek.*

The Deer Creek Trail soon emerges into Deer Creek Valley, where there are plenty of campsites.

Follow the Deer Creek Trail east up the slope. Deer Spring, to the right of the trail, marks the noisy source of Deer Creek. After the spring, the trail climbs up a canyon below the towering Redwall limestone cliff, and finally emerges onto the west rim of Surprise Valley, where it meets the Thunder River Trail.

Turn left (north) on the Thunder River Trail. Numerous switchbacks ascend a rockslide that makes this route through the Redwall limestone and Supai formation possible. Once on the Esplanade, follow the Thunder River Trail east toward Bridger Knoll and then north along the Esplanade. As you pass west of Monument Point, the Monument Point Trail branches right. Stay left on the original Thunder River Trail, which continues along the Esplanade. The trail is at the head of the many forks of Deer Creek where it splits north and west. As it approaches a point below Little Saddle, the trail starts to climb the talus slope. Here you pass the point where you left the trail, closing the loop. Continue over Little Saddle and on to the Indian Hollow Trailhead.

Tip: *The following itinerary should be considered a minimum, and 9 or 10 days would not be an excessive time to spend on this trip.*

POSSIBLE ITINERARY

	Camp	Miles	Elevation Gain
Day 1	Indian Hollow	6.5	700
Day 2	Mountain Sheep Spring	6.5	0
Day 3	Kanab Canyon	7.0	0
Day 4	Kanab Canyon	7.0	0
Day 5	Colorado River	7.0	0
Day 6	Deer Creek	6.8	920
Day 7	Out	11.4	3950

SCOTTY'S HOLLOW OPTIONAL SIDE HIKE You'll find numerous side canyons to explore along Kanab Creek, and one of the most popular is Scotty's Hollow. Though not labeled on the U.S.G.S. topographic map, it's the first canyon on the right (west) side of Kanab Creek downstream of Showerbath Spring.

WHISPERING FALLS OPTIONAL SIDE HIKE Another interesting side canyon is on the left (east) side of Kanab Creek, several miles south of Scotty's Hollow. A steep chute a short distance up this canyon forms a waterfall informally known as Whispering Falls.

THUNDER RIVER OPTIONAL SIDE HIKE From the junction of the Deer Creek Trail and the Thunder River Trail, go right (east) on the Thunder River Trail. The heavily used trail leads past the east rim of Surprise Valley, where you immediately hear the roar of Thunder Spring. Thunder River—the shortest river in the world—cascades half a mile to join Tapeats Creek.

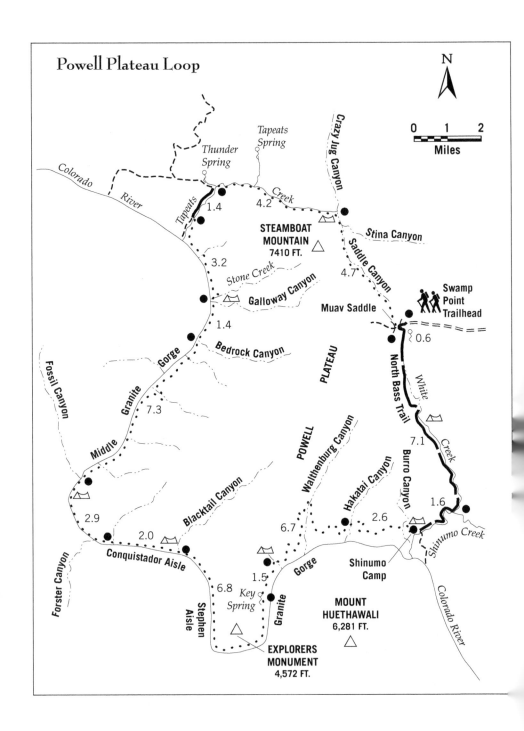

Powell Plateau Loop

N

Colorado River

Thunder Spring

Tapeats Spring

Crazy Jug Canyon

0   1   2
Miles

1.4   Tapeats   Creek   4.2

STEAMBOAT MOUNTAIN 7410 FT.

Stina Canyon

Saddle Canyon   4.7

Swamp Point Trailhead

3.2

Stone Creek   Galloway Canyon

Muav Saddle

0.6

1.4

PLATEAU

North Bass Trail

White

Bedrock Canyon

Fossil Canyon

Granite   Gorge   7.3

Creek

7.1

Middle

POWELL

Walthenburg Canyon

Hakatai Canyon

Burro Canyon

1.6

2.9

Blacktail Canyon

6.7

2.6

Shinumo Creek

2.0

Conquistador Aisle

Forster Canyon

Gorge

Shinumo Camp

Colorado River

1.5

6.8   Key Spring

Granite

MOUNT HUETHAWALI 6,281 FT.

Stephen Aisle

EXPLORERS MONUMENT 4,572 FT.

RATINGS (1–10)			MILES	ELEVATION GAIN	DAYS	SHUTTLE MILEAGE
Scenery	Solitude	Difficulty	54.6	7250	9	0
10	10	10				

MAPS King Arthur Castle, Tapeats Amphitheater, Powell Plateau, Fossil Bay, Topocoba Hilltop, Explorers Monument, Havasupai Point U.S.G.S.

SEASON Mid September–November.

BEST October.

WATER Muav Saddle Spring, Tapeats Creek, Colorado River, Key Spring, Hakatai Canyon, Shinumo Creek, and White Creek.

PERMITS Required for camping within Grand Canyon National Park.

RULES Campfires are not allowed in the national park backcountry. Pets are not allowed on trails or in the backcountry.

CONTACT Grand Canyon National Park, P.O. Box 129, Grand Canyon, Arizona 86023, (928) 638-7888, www.nps.gov/grca.

HIGHLIGHTS This is an especially scenic and remote loop around Powell Plateau along the Colorado River. Several permanent streams grace the route, including Thunder River, Shinumo Creek, and White Creek. You'll spend days hiking along the Colorado River's banks, or along the top of cliffs a few hundred feet above the Colorado River. The loop takes you through Middle Granite Gorge, Conquistador Aisle, Stephen Aisle, and Granite Gorge. You'll find plenty of side canyons to explore, including Stone, Galloway, Bedrock, and Blacktail canyons.

PROBLEMS This is a strenuous cross-country hike. All members of the party should be fit, and the leader should have experience hiking cross-country in the Grand Canyon. Those without such experience should choose one of the on-trail Grand Canyon hikes—Tanner Trail to Kaibab Trail, or South Bass Trail to Hermit Trail. You must have the U.S.G.S. 7.5 minute topographic maps for critical route finding on this hike.

Warning: Do not underestimate the difficulty of this hike. Your rate of progress may average one mile per hour, and can fall to half a mile per hour at times. Map miles do not accurately reflect hiking distances in the Grand Canyon because of the rough terrain. Additionally, this hike is dangerous during the summer. Do not attempt it from May through mid September, when temperatures commonly exceed 100°F.

Tip: Bring a 50-foot, 6 or 7 mm rope for hauling packs.

Water sources are often far apart, and each hiker should have enough water containers to carry water for an overnight dry camp.

HOW TO GET THERE From Jacob Lake at the junction of U.S. 89A and Arizona 67, drive 26.8 miles south on Arizona 67, and then turn right (west) on Forest Road 22. At the top of the hill, after 2.1 miles, turn left (south) on Forest Road 270. Drive 2.2 miles and turn right on Forest Road 223. Continue 5.3 miles; turn left (south) on Forest Road 268. After about 0.5 mile, turn left on Forest Road 268B.

Warning: This road is snowed in during the winter. Major snowstorms can come any time from November through March, and the road is normally impassable into May or June.

Now comes the tricky part—Forest Road 268B heads south and crosses into Grand Canyon National Park, but a confusing maze of logging roads has been built north of the park boundary. You will have to try each left spur until you find the road that continues through the unmarked park gate. Just beyond this gate, you'll reach the Kanabonits Road junction. Turn right (west) onto the Swamp Point Road, and continue 7.2 miles to the end of the road at the Swamp Point Trailhead.

DESCRIPTION Descend into the Grand Canyon via the North Bass Trail, which switchbacks down into Muav Saddle, the broad pass separating Powell Plateau from the North Rim. Just as you reach Muav Saddle, an unmarked spur trail goes south to an unnamed spring at the base of the buff Coconino sandstone. A few yards further along, the North Bass Trail also branches left: this is the return route. Stay right on the main trail across Muav Saddle, and look for

Geologic faults in the rocks create most of the routes followed by hikers and trail builders through the cliffs of the Grand Canyon. The beginning and end of this loop are made possible by the Muav Fault, which cuts through Muav Saddle from south to north. Along this fault, rocks are lifted higher on one side than on the other, fracturing the horizontal layers of rock. Erosion takes advantage of this shattered rock to carve out side canyons and breaks through cliffs. The cross-country descent along Saddle Canyon follows the Muav Fault, as does the North Bass Trail in White Canyon.

a spur trail on the right (north). Take this unnamed trail 100 yards to Theodore Roosevelt's Cabin.

To start the loop section of the trip, hike cross-country down Saddle Canyon north of the cabin. Much of the area north of Muav Saddle is covered with thick oak brush as the result of a series of wildfires. The bed of Saddle Canyon is the easiest route. You'll find no major obstacles until you reach a high fall in the reddish Supai formation 2.4 miles below Muav Saddle, at the 5800-foot contour. Bypass the fall by following a cairned route to the west, and down the ridge west of the bed. The route returns to the bed of Saddle Canyon for just 0.3 mile before reaching the start of the Redwall limestone gorge. Bypass a fall at the start of the gorge via a fault route to the west. Several chockstones in the bed present minor obstacles. Further in the Redwall descent, you'll encounter the Slicky Slide, a narrow chute leading down to a pool. Descend the polished limestone chute with care by straddling the small stream that usually flows down the middle. The cold pool of water at the bottom has to be waded.

Tip: Make note of the route the first person uses, because mud stirred up from the bottom will make it impossible for the rest of the party to see the deep areas.

Bypass the high fall at the base of the Redwall on a game trail to the left (west). Stina Canyon comes in from the right, and there are campsites here and at the head of Tapeats Creek, where Crazy Jug Canyon comes in from the north. You'll find campsites downstream along Tapeats Creek.

Continue downstream (west) along Tapeats Creek. The flow in upper Tapeats Creek is normally low and the going is easy until you reach the unnamed side canyon from the north that contains Tapeats Spring. This spring contributes most of the water to Tapeats Creek, and below this side canyon a narrows formed in the Tapeats sandstone requires you to wade the racing, foot-deep water at several points. A walking stick can be useful here.

After the narrows end, you'll come to Thunder River, a boisterous tributary entering from the west. Thunder River offers an optional side hike.

Continue the main loop by following the informal trail down the right (west) side of Tapeats Creek. The trail crosses Tapeats Creek several times, but ultimately returns to the right bank. At the 2200-foot contour, where a gorge starts to form, leave the trail and cross Tapeats Creek . Follow a fainter river-runners trail along narrow terraces on the left side of Tapeats Creek Canyon. This trail contours above the lower gorge of Tapeats Creek, and then rounds the point above the Colorado River and heads southeast. The informal trail makes for easy walking past Hundred and Thirty-three Mile Creek to Stone Creek. Follow Stone Creek to the Colorado River, where there are campsites. Stone Creek offers an optional side hike.

Follow the Colorado River upstream (south) past Galloway Canyon. South of Galloway Canyon, riverside cliffs will force you to climb up above the Colorado River several times, depending on the Colorado River's flow. Bedrock Canyon provides access to the river and good campsites.

Tip: *Glen Canyon Dam, upstream above the park, controls the Colorado River, and the Colorado River's level varies on a daily cycle according to the amount of power being generated at the dam.*

South of Bedrock Canyon, the deepening Middle Granite Gorge forces you to climb the point between the Colorado River and Bedrock Canyon. You'll need to work your way to the terrace at the top of the purplish-brown Tapeats sandstone, at the 2600-foot level, before you reach the next side canyon upstream. Old burro trails make the going relatively easy along this terrace. At Hundred and Twentyeight Mile Creek you'll have to detour around the side canyon's lower gorge. Seasonal water flows where you cross the bed of Hundred and Twentyeight Mile Creek. From the crossing, follow the bed to the Colorado River where campsites are limited.

To continue the hike upriver from the mouth of Hundred and Twenty-eight Mile Creek, you'll have to climb above the Tapeats

🦎 Wild Burros

Wild burros, which came from animals brought in by prospectors, are excellent trail makers. Though the Park Service was forced to remove or shoot the burros in the 1970s, their nicely contoured trails remain and are used by the occasional backpacker. The burros had to go because they were competing with the native desert bighorn sheep. The sheep have since increased their range—watch for these stately animals throughout this hike.

sandstone and remain at this level to the upper end of Middle Granite Gorge. Descend to the Colorado River at Fossil Rapids opposite the mouth of Fossil Canyon. You can continue upstream along the left bank, except for a couple of short, nasty bypasses where you'll have to climb up and across outcroppings of sharp travertine rock.

Though tedious, the travertine section is soon past, and you're rewarded by several stretches of sidewalk-like walking provided by ledges of Tapeats sandstone exposed at river level. Campsites are plentiful and the going easy as you follow the Colorado River upstream past the mouth of Forster Canyon and east into Conquistador Aisle. East of Hundred and Twentytwo Mile Creek, you'll have to climb to the top of the Tapeats sandstone to continue upstream 1.9 miles to Blacktail Canyon. Blacktail Canyon offers easy access to riverside campsites.

This is a good spot to spend the night before tackling the long section ahead, where you'll be walking along the top of the Tapeats sandstone cliff, several hundred feet above the Colorado River. Water is scarce along this terrace and river access limited by the persistent Tapeats cliff below you. Two routes lead to the Colorado River before Key Spring, but these may be difficult to find.

Warning: *It is 6.8 miles to the next reliable water source at Key Spring.*

In cool weather, you can expect to find water pockets in some of the side canyons as you continue upstream from Blacktail Canyon along the Tapeats sandstone terrace.

Tip: *Search up and downstream from your point of crossing for these pockets of rainwater collected in potholes in the bedrock.*

As the Colorado River turns north, the inner gorge becomes deeper as the ancient Precambrian rocks become exposed. A spring

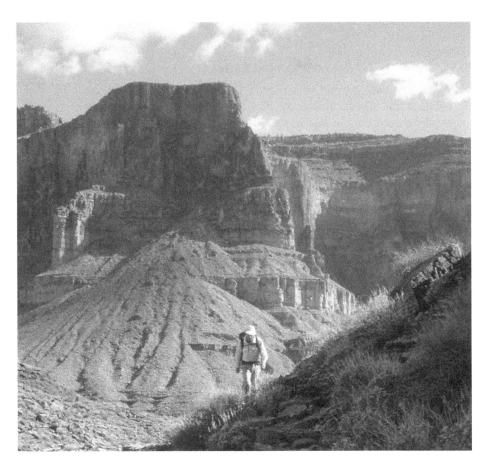

Hiking into Walthenberg Canyon

discovered by George Steck is located in a side canyon 0.4 mile north-east of the 4850T elevation point on the topographic map. George named this water source Key Spring, since it makes a long, waterless stretch much less dangerous.

The loop continues north along the Tapeats sandstone rim, and the going becomes slower as you are forced to contour around a deep, nameless side canyon. Contouring around Walthenburg Canyon is especially slow, though there are campsites and seasonal water pockets in the second of its westside canyons. East of Walthenburg Canyon, follow the top of the Tapeats around toward Hakatai Canyon.

Here you enter the region explored by William Bass at the end of the nineteenth century. Bass built several trails and mines, and later guided tourists into the Grand Canyon along his North and South Bass trails. The two trails were connected by a low water ferry, and by two aerial tram cables for use during the spring floods.

A trace of one of Bass's trails helps you on the descent into Hakatai Canyon. Descend south in the last shallow drainage before reaching Hakatai Canyon, and you'll pick up a faint trail leading around the point between Hakatai and the Colorado River. The trail then descends north-northeast into the bed of Hakatai. An optional side hike leads down Hakatai Canyon to the Colorado River.

The main loop continues cross-country east out of Hakatai Canyon, up the prominent ravine almost directly toward Fan Island. Contour south of Fan Island on the terrace above the Tapeats sandstone. You may pick up traces of Bass's old trail connecting Hakatai Canyon to his main camp at Shinumo Creek as you proceed. Descend east into Burro Canyon along a ramp located 0.5 mile southeast of Fan Island. The route goes below the rim of Burro Canyon, and descends a talus slope directly to the bed. Climb east out of Burro Canyon and over the ridge separating it from Shinumo Creek; descend east to meet the creek where the topographic map shows the North Bass Trail descending to the creek from the south side. It's a short walk upstream along the North Bass Trail to Shinumo Camp. Though several major floods have ravaged the area since Bass abandoned it, there are still artifacts remaining from his time in the Grand Canyon. Campsites are plentiful, and the rushing waters of Shinumo Creek are a delight.

Follow the North Bass Trail up Shinumo Creek. Although the King Arthur Castle topographic map shows the main trail leaving the creek and climbing a slope to the north, this section is badly eroded and very rough. It's much easier and more enjoyable to follow the hiker's trail on up Shinumo Creek. Turn left (north) into White Creek. The canyon enters an impressive narrows in the Tapeats sandstone north of Redwall Canyon, and you'll spot a huge chockstone jammed high between the walls. A fall blocks the upper end of the gorge, but there is an easy route out on the right. Above the Tapeats, you'll rejoin the North Bass Trail, which generally follows the dry bed of the wash on up Muav Canyon, except where it leaves the bed to bypass obstacles. As the Redwall limestone cliffs close in above you, water surfaces in the bed, and this is a possible area to camp before the final ascent to the rim.

▲▲▲ Granite Gorges

Access to the Colorado River along the river section of the loop is controlled by the geology of the rocks exposed along the river. Since the best way to hike this loop is counterclockwise, you'll be hiking upstream along the Colorado River. The geology along the river was first described by Major John Wesley Powell on his pioneering Colorado River trip in 1869. You'll encounter features in the opposite order of his account. At the mouth of Tapeats Creek, the Tapeats sandstone is exposed at river level. This resistant sandstone forms a cliff about 200 feet high, pieces of which often fall directly into the river, making it impossible to walk the bank upstream. The only practical hiking route is along the top of the Tapeats sandstone, where a sloping terrace is formed on the soft, easily eroded Bright Angel shale. Called the Tonto Plateau, this terrace makes the low level loop around Powell Plateau possible. Breaks in the Tapeats sandstone at Stone and Galloway canyons provide access routes to the Colorado River. As you hike upstream past Galloway Canyon, the dark gray Vishnu schist starts to appear at river level, marking the lower end of Middle Granite Gorge. This ancient, resistant rock erodes into a steep, V-shaped gorge, rimmed by the 200-foot brownish cliffs of the Tapeats sandstone. Pinkish intrusions of granite occur in the Vishnu schist, thus the name Middle Granite Gorge.

The presence of various layers of rock at Colorado River level is controlled by the general level of the Colorado Plateau. Different sections of the plateau have been lifted to various elevations, so the river encounters a succession of rock layers as it meanders across the Colorado Plateau. The Vishnu schist is exposed at three major locations along the Colorado River's course as it meanders through the Grand Canyon. At each of these three places, deep, steep-walled inner gorges are formed. The upstream gorge, the first encountered by Major Powell, was named simply, Granite Gorge. The second and third gorges are Middle and Lower Granite Gorges.

At Fossil Rapids, the Vishnu schist disappears below river level, marking the upper end of Middle Granite Gorge. A few ledges of Tapeats sandstone are exposed, but the soft Bright Angel shale largely determines the topography along the river banks. It's possible to hike the bank for several miles, until the Tapeats sandstone reappears at Hundred and Twentytwo Mile Canyon. Throughout Conquistador and Stephen Aisles, the Tapeats sandstone forms a sheer gorge along the Colorado River, and access to the river from the route along the Tonto Plateau is severely limited by the steep cliffs. Access gets rarer upstream of Stephen Aisle, where the Vishnu schist reappears. This marks the lower end of Granite Gorge, which rapidly grows deeper as you proceed north past Walthenburg Canyon. At Hakatai Canyon, the steep terrain is relived somewhat by the appearance of the Grand Canyon series of rocks. Formed of tilted layers of sandstone, shale, and quartzite, the Grand Canyon series is found on top of the Vishnu schist and below the Tapeats sandstone, so its presence creates a few slopes and dipping terraces in the otherwise cliff-bound Granite Gorge.

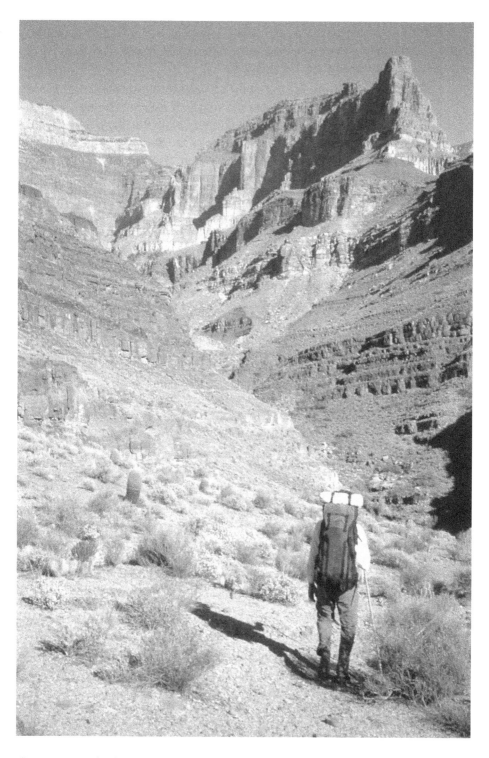

Cross-country backpacking below Powell Plateau

Tip: This is the last reliable water before Muav Saddle. Campsites are also scarce after the Redwall ascent.

Watch carefully for the point where the North Bass Trail leaves the bed on the left and starts the Redwall ascent. The trail switchbacks its way up this unlikely looking break in the massive cliffs, and then works its way along the west rim of the Redwall gorge before returning to the bed of upper Muav Canyon. At the head of the canyon, the old trail climbs steeply up the reddish Supai formation slopes to Muav Saddle, closing the loop. Turn right and hike the North Bass Trail to the trailhead.

Tip: The following itinerary should be considered a minimum, and 12 days would not be an excessive time to spend on this trip.

POSSIBLE ITINERARY

	Camp	Miles	Elevation Gain
Day 1	Tapeats Creek	7.3	0
Day 2	Stone Creek	6.8	0
Day 3	Bedrock Canyon	1.4	200
Day 4	Fossil Canyon	7.3	400
Day 5	Blacktail Canyon	4.9	200
Day 6	Key Spring	8.3	480
Day 7	Shinumo Creek	9.3	980
Day 8	White Creek	5.1	2000
Day 9	Out	4.2	2990

THUNDER RIVER OPTIONAL SIDE HIKE An informal trail follows Thunder River upstream 0.5 mile to a point opposite Thunder Springs, its source. All of the water in Thunder River comes from this single spring.

STONE CREEK OPTIONAL SIDE HIKE You can hike cross-country upstream following Stone Creek 2.0 miles to a pretty waterfall in the Tapeats sandstone.

COLORADO RIVER OPTIONAL SIDE HIKE An obscure cross-country route to the Colorado River in Stephen Aisle is located just south of the southernmost unnamed rapids on the 7.5 minute topographic map, on the east bank of the Colorado River. Watch below for a large terrace in the Tapeats sandstone that is sunk below the general rim level. This terrace is big enough for a campsite in a pinch, and there's a route to the Colorado River via ledges at its north end. This route is primarily useful for getting water if you haven't been able to find any along the Tapeats rim or in side drainages.

EXPLORERS MONUMENT OPTIONAL SIDE HIKE After the Colorado River turns east around Explorers Monument, there is another route to the Colorado River. An unnamed drainage starts east of Explorers Monument and drops into the Colorado River. The route descends just west of this drainage, south of the 2532T elevation point on the Explorers Monument topographic map. This route is primarily useful to get water. If you do need water here, it would probably be easier to camp on the top of the Tapeats sandstone, and do a side hike to the Colorado River for water.

5140T OPTIONAL SIDE HIKE Another route to the Colorado River goes down the nameless side canyon 0.8 mile east-northeast of the 5140T elevation point. Again, it would be easiest to leave your packs on the top of the Tapeats and side hike to the Colorado River for water.

> *Tip:* Look for water pockets in the bed below the point where you cross it, before heading to the Colorado River for water.

The route to the Colorado River follows the bed two-thirds of the way, and then veers out to the right (south) to avoid a dry waterfall. Work your way east down the rocky slope south of the main drainage to reach the Colorado River's edge. This side hike is worth doing even if you don't need water.

HAKATAI CANYON OPTIONAL SIDE HIKE Hike down the bed of Hakatai Canyon from the point where you reached it. Just before you reach the Colorado River, watch for a trail up a steep ravine on the left. This spur trail leads to a platform that anchored one end of Bass's Hakatai Cable. The view up and down river from the old cable terminus is spectacular. Look carefully at the slope on the far side of the Colorado River, and you can spot the trail to the other terminus of the tramway. The cable itself was removed in the 1970s as a potential hazard to river boats.

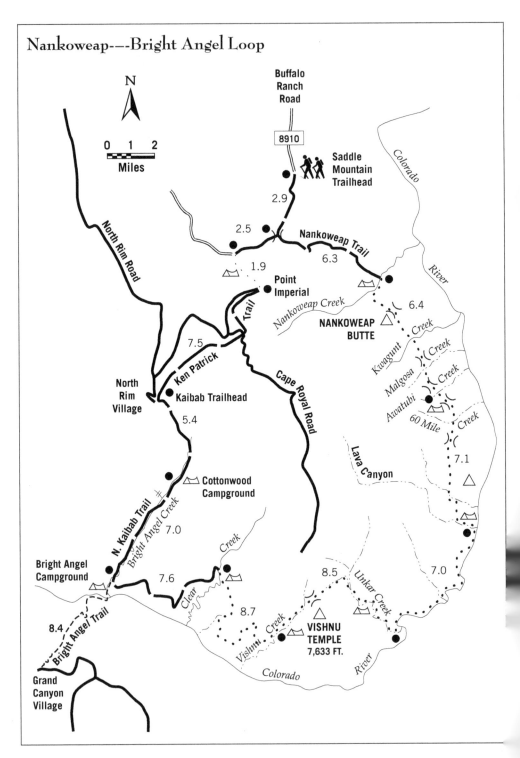

Nankoweap---Bright Angel Loop

Buffalo Ranch Road

8910

Saddle Mountain Trailhead

2.9

2.5

Nankoweap Trail

6.3

North Rim Road

1.9

Point Imperial

Trail

Nankoweap Creek

6.4

NANKOWEAP BUTTE

Kwagunt Creek

7.5

Ken Patrick

Malgosa Creek

North Rim Village

Kaibab Trailhead

Cape Royal Road

Avatubi

60 Mile Creek

5.4

7.1

Lava Canyon

Cottonwood Campground

N. Kaibab Trail

Bright Angel Creek

7.0

Creek

7.0

Bright Angel Campground

7.6

8.5

Unkar Creek

8.4

Bright Angel Trail

Clear

8.7

Vishnu Creek

VISHNU TEMPLE 7,633 FT.

Grand Canyon Village

Colorado River

N

0 1 2
Miles

Colorado River

7 Nankoweap–Bright Angel Loop

RATINGS (1–10)			MILES	ELEVATION GAIN	DAYS	SHUTTLE MILEAGE
Scenery	Solitude	Difficulty	82.2	16,830	11	0
10	10	10	(63.7)	(14,190)	(10)	(179)

MAPS Point Imperial, Nankoweap Mesa, Bright Angel Point, Phantom Ranch U.S.G.S.

SEASON Mid September–May.

BEST October–November, March–April.

WATER Nankoweap Creek, Kwagunt Creek, Colorado River, Unkar Creek, seasonally in Vishnu Creek, Clear Creek, Bright Angel Creek.

PERMITS Required for camping within Grand Canyon National Park.

RULES Campfires are not allowed in the national park backcountry. Along the North Kaibab Trail near the end of the loop, camping is only allowed in designated campgrounds. Pets are not allowed on trails or in the backcountry.

CONTACT Grand Canyon National Park, P.O. Box 129, Grand Canyon, Arizona 86023, (928) 638-7888, www.nps.gov/grca.

HIGHLIGHTS This scenic loop takes you through spectacular geology of the eastern Grand Canyon, past permanent streams and towering, cliff-bound buttes and mesas. In the eastern Grand Canyon, colorful layers of the Grand Canyon series of rock formations meet the somber, ancient metamorphic rocks of the Granite Gorge, creating a dramatic change in the shape of the Grand Canyon's floor. Most of this loop is seldom traveled and you're unlikely to meet any other hikers on the cross-country section of the loop.

PROBLEMS This is a strenuous cross-country hike. All members of the party should be fit, and the leader should have experience hiking cross-country in the Grand Canyon. Those without such experience should choose one of the on-trail Grand Canyon hikes—Tanner Trail to Kaibab Trail, or South Bass Trail to Hermit Trail. You must have the U.S.G.S. 7.5 minute topographic maps for critical route finding on this hike. Water sources are often far apart, and each hiker should have enough water containers to carry water for an overnight dry camp. If you do this hike in the spring, before the North Rim is open, you'll have to use the optional South Rim exit, via the Bright Angel trail. This requires that you leave a vehicle at the Bright Angel Trailhead in Grand Canyon Village. This hike is dangerous during the summer. Do not attempt it from May through mid September, when temperatures commonly exceed 100°F.

Warning: Do not underestimate the difficulty of this hike. Your rate of progress may average one mile per hour, and can fall to half a mile per hour at times. Map miles do not accurately reflect hiking distances in the Grand Canyon because of the rough terrain.

Tip: Bring a 50-foot, 6 or 7 mm rope for hauling packs. You'll encounter several places where hikers may require a rope belay for safety.

HOW TO GET THERE From Flagstaff, drive 111 miles north on U.S. 89 and turn left (north) on U.S. 89A. Continue 14 miles to Marble Canyon; drive another 21.6 miles to the Buffalo Ranch Road. Turn left (south) on this dirt road, and continue 27.0 miles to its end at the Saddle Mountain Trailhead. This road may be impassable in winter, or after a major winter storm.

To reach the Bright Angel Trailhead from Cameron on U.S. 89, drive 52 miles west on Arizona 64, to Grand Canyon Village. The trailhead is at the west end of the village, near Bright Angel Lodge.

DESCRIPTION Start out on the Saddle Mountain Trail, which heads south and climbs up a gradual ridge through the pinyon pine and juniper forest. In 1.0 mile the Saddle Mountain Trail swings east and drops into Saddle Canyon, where it meets the Nankoweap Trail. Turn right and follow the Nankoweap Trail south up the bed of Saddle Canyon. As Saddle Canyon opens out into a forested basin, the trail leaves the drainage and follows a ridge south, uphill, through fine stands of ponderosa pine.

When the trail reaches Boundary Ridge, 2.9 miles from the trailhead, it meets the original upper section of the Nankoweap Trail, which comes from the North Rim of the Grand Canyon, to your west.

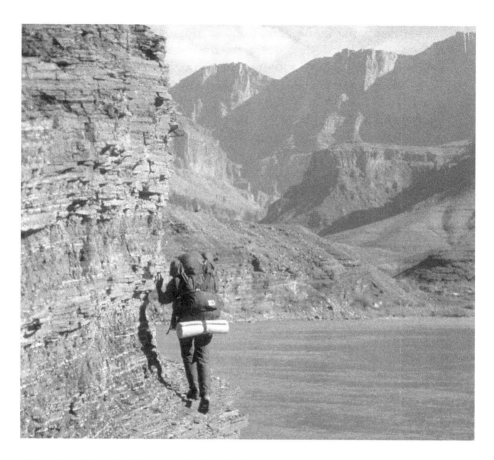

Above the Colorado River near Unkar Creek

This is the return route. Turn left (east) and follow the Nankoweap Trail down into the unnamed saddle west of Saddle Mountain. From here, the Nankoweap Trail descends the upper sandstone cliffs of the Supai formation in a series of short switchbacks.

> **Warning:** *You'll encounter a bad section of trail before it rounds Point 6961. A section of the original trail construction has fallen away, and the tread traverses a steep shale slope above a cliff. While not a problem if the trail is dry, this section can be dangerous if the ground is muddy. A rope belay may be required.*

Once below this cliff band, it stays at this level in the Supai formation, heading generally east. As the Nankoweap Trail continues east along the tilted Supai formation ledges, it steadily loses elevation.

Eventually, the trail emerges onto a ridge and descends onto the west rim of Tilted Mesa. Here, the trail turns south and descends a broken slope trough the Redwall limestone formation to reach gentle shale slopes that lead southeast to Nankoweap Creek, where the trail ends, 6.3 miles from Boundary Ridge. Perennial Nankoweap Creek is graced with Fremont cottonwood trees, and campsites are plentiful. An optional cross-country side hike follows lower Nankoweap Creek to the Colorado River.

South of Nankoweap Creek, the route follows a route commonly referred to as the Horse Thief Trail. Since there probably never was a constructed trail along this route, and there is little trace of a trail today, I'll refer to it as the Horse Thief Route. Head southwest up Nankoweap Creek, and turn left up an unnamed drainage toward Nankoweap Butte. The going is easy through the pygmy pinyon pine and juniper forest, and you can cross the divide between Nankoweap and Kwagunt creeks on either side of Nankoweap Butte.

▲▲ East Kaibab Monocline

The Horse Thief Route is made possible by the Butte Fault and the East Kaibab Monocline. Although there is some evidence that thieves did use the route to move stolen animals from Arizona to Utah, there never was a constructed trail along the route. Probably used mostly by prospectors, a few horseshoes and other artifacts are the only evidence that suggests this was ever a well-traveled route. A monocline sometimes forms when one block of horizontal rock layers is uplifted higher than the adjoining block. In the process, the rock layers flow like toothpaste, tilting steeply along the boundary. In the case of the East Kaibab Monocline, the rocks to the west have been lifted about 3000 feet higher than the rocks to the east. The formerly horizontal sedimentary layers along the monocline have been tilted to the vertical. There has also been vertical slippage along the Butte Fault in places, which shatters the rocks. Erosion forms side canyons along the fault and monocline, and the Horse Thief Route takes advantage of these small canyons to find a way across Nankoweap, Kwagunt, Malgosa, Awatubi, 60 Mile, and Carbon creeks. The East Kaibab Monocline continues far to the north and south of the Grand Canyon—in fact, it's the longest exposed monocline on the planet.

Descend into the unnamed drainages south of the butte, and head for Kwagunt Creek at a point upstream (west) of the Butte Fault. This massive fault is marked by formerly horizontal rock layers now tilted vertical. The Butte Fault is clearly visible just to the west of the vertical rocks, where the fault zone erodes into small canyons that cross the main canyons, such as Kwagunt Creek, at right angles. From the saddles on either side of Nankoweap Butte, you can clearly see the gray and red ramparts of tilted Redwall limestone on either side of Kwagunt Creek. This is the same formation you encountered on the Nankoweap Trail, thousands of feet higher. Follow the drainage system down to Kwagunt Creek, 3.5 miles from Nankoweap Creek. Kwagunt Creek has a small perennial flow. An optional cross-country side hike follows Kwagunt Creek 2.5 miles east to the Colorado River.

Tip: Pick up water at Kwagunt Creek for a dry camp, as there are no permanent water sources along the remainder of the Horse Thief Route.

From Kwagunt Creek, hike south up the nameless canyon just west of the Butte Fault. You'll need to do some some minor route finding to avoid small cliffs, especially near the saddle at the canyon's head. From the saddle, continue down to Malgosa Creek via the ravine just east of the fault. Malgosa Creek is 1.4 miles from Kwagunt Creek. Malgosa Creek is normally dry at the Horse Thief Route crossing, though you may find water by walking downstream. In a pinch, you can hike east down Malgosa Creek to the Colorado River, but Malgosa Creek is much harder than Nankoweap and Kwagunt Creeks.

Cross the pass west of Kwagunt Butte and descend to Awatubi Creek via the ravines just west of the Butte Fault. Awatubi Creek is

1.4 miles from Malgosa Creek. Awatubi Creek is normally dry where the route crosses, but you may be able to find water downstream. Awatubi Creek cannot be followed to the Colorado River. A seasonal water source is a series of deep water pockets in the sandstone terraces northeast of Awatubi Crest, though this is 0.8 mile off the route. You'll find small campsites in Awatubi Creek near the Horse Thief Route crossing.

~~~ Peaking Power and Grand Canyon Routes

The amount of water released by Glen Canyon Dam now controls the level of the Colorado River. Since hydroelectric power generated at the dam is used to meet peak power needs, the amount of power used in distant cities determines the amount of water released. Power use peaks on a daily basis as air conditioners are switched on during the hot part of the day. A daily pattern of rising and falling water throughout the length of the Colorado River is evident in the Grand Canyon. The level changes as much as five feet every day. At low water, it is possible to walk the right bank of the river from Tanner Rapids to Unkar Rapids. If the water is high, small cliff bands may block the route. If you have a few hours to spare, you may wait for lower water and avoid a detour along the bluffs above the cliffs.

To continue, follow the ravine to the saddle just west of Awatubi Crest, and then down the fault ravine on the south side into a nameless side canyon of 60 Mile Creek. Climb over a minor saddle and descend into the main branch of the creek, 1.4 miles from Awatubi Creek. 60 Mile Creek is normally dry, and there is no route to the Colorado River. You'll find plenty of camping along 60 Mile Creek at the Horse Thief Route Crossing.

South of 60 Mile Creek, climb the westernmost of the two canyons that climb to the south, and pass over the saddle west of Chuar Butte to reach the East Fork Carbon Creek. Now, descend the East Fork Carbon Creek to the south, bypassing the small cliff bands as needed.

Tip: Carbon Creek is normally dry, but the Colorado River is easy to reach via the lower canyon.

Exactly 0.5 mile after the canyon turns east, and 3.6 miles from 60 Mile Creek, leave Carbon Creek and head south 0.9 mile over a low saddle into Lava Creek. Head downstream, and follow Lava Canyon 1.0 mile to the Colorado River and the end of the Horse Thief Route. You'll find several campsites at the mouth of the canyon.

Follow the right bank of the Colorado River downstream. Cross the unnamed drainage 0.8 mile south of Lava Creek; leave the Colorado River and climb the ridge to the southwest toward Point 4201.

Tip: It is normally impossible to continue at river level because of cliff bands that drop directly into the Colorado River, though it has been done at very low water.

Just below the top of Point 4201, head south along the east-facing slopes. The shale slope is uncomfortably steep, and the higher you climb, the less of this nasty traverse you'll have to cross. Ideally, you'll have about half a mile of traversing to reach the ridge south-southeast of Point 4201. Descend this ridge, cross an unnamed drainage, and follow the rim of the cliff above the Colorado River until you can descend to the broad gravel bar just upstream of Tanner Rapids. Now, follow the right bank of the Colorado River 4.6 miles downstream to Unkar Creek. You'll find several small cliff bands that may have to be bypassed at high water. Campsites are plentiful on the open expanse of Unkar Delta.

Continue the route by hiking up Unkar Creek. Water usually surfaces about two miles upstream from the Colorado River, and there are several possible campsites. At the 3800-foot contour, 3.8 miles from the Colorado River, turn left into an unnamed fork of Unkar Creek. This fork remains parallel to Unkar Creek for 0.6 mile, heading north, before turning abruptly southwest toward the nameless saddle between Vishnu Temple and Freya Castle. Head up this canyon for 0.5 mile, then leave the bed to the south to bypass a high fall in the Tapeats sandstone. Above the fall, rejoin the bed of the drainage for the rest of the climb to the saddle. You'll find one tricky section near the top of the Redwall limestone, where you will probably want to pass packs or haul them with a rope. The Vishnu–Freya saddle is 2.4 miles from the fork in Unkar Creek.

Descend southwest down the unnamed side canyon into Vishnu Creek. You will probably need to pass packs or lower them on a rope at two chockstones on this descent, and some members of the party may need a rope belay.

Tip: Watch for a small spring on the left as you descend the greenish Muav formation below the Redwall limestone. This is a good alternate water source in the event there's none in Vishnu Creek.

You may find seasonal water in Vishnu Creek above the point where the bed descends into the brownish Tapeats sandstone. You'll find several campsites above the 4000-foot contour in Vishnu Creek, 2.2 miles from the Vishnu–Freya saddle.

The cross-country route continues west of Vishnu Creek on the Tonto Plateau, the terrace above the Tapeats sandstone. Leave Vishnu Creek on about the 4000-foot contour, walk around Hall Butte, and cross the nameless canyon to the west, where you may find seasonal water pockets in the bed of the drainage. After you swing around Hawkins Butte, you'll spot The Howlands Butte to the north. The route goes over the unnamed saddle to the east of The Howlands Butte, and then drops north into Clear Creek via a nameless tributary. It may take some searching to find the descent through the Tapeats sandstone from above, but after that the route is not difficult to Clear Creek and its delightful perennial stream. It is 8.2 miles from Vishnu Creek to Clear Creek. You'll find plenty of campsites along Clear Creek.

Head upstream 0.5 mile to the unnamed side canyon joining Clear Creek from the left (northwest). Go up this side canyon 0.1 mile to find the start of the Clear Creek Trail, which climbs the side canyon wall to the south. The Clear Creek Trail, though not maintained, is frequently used and is in relatively good shape. Ascend the trail through the Tapeats sandstone and onto the Tonto Plateau, and then contour around Zoroaster Canyon before turning west toward Sumner Point. You may find seasonal water pockets in the bed of the nameless canyon just east of Sumner Point. South of the point, the trail descends through the Tapeats sandstone before turning north and descending into Bright Angel Canyon. The Clear Creek Trail ends at the heavily used North Kaibab Trail, 7.6 miles from Clear Creek. The optional Bright Angel Trail south rim exit goes left here.

To continue on the main loop from the junction with the Clear Creek Trail, turn right (north) on the North Kaibab Trail, which follows Bright Angel Creek through The Box. You'll soon pass the impressive mouth of Phantom Canyon. Precisely 6.0 miles from the Clear Creek Trail, watch for the 0.3-mile spur trail to pretty Ribbon Falls on the west side of the canyon. Back on the North Kaibab Trail,

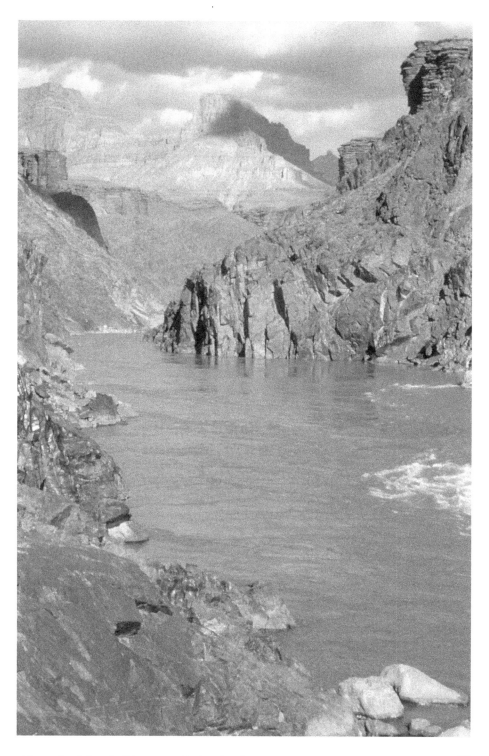

Along the Colorado River near Unkar Creek

≈ Snowmelt Floods on the Colorado River

Before Glen Canyon Dam was finished in 1964, the Colorado River reached its annual high stage in the Grand Canyon during early summer, when snowmelt from the distant Rocky Mountains reached the canyons. One such spring flood in the 1880's crested at 300,000 cubic feet per second, as measured by the location of driftwood left high above the river's normal banks. At the mouth of Clear Creek, driftwood from this event is about 100 feet above the present river level.

you'll reach Cottonwood Camp 1.0 mile from the Ribbons Falls Trail. At the mouth of Manzanita Canyon, the trail passes a ranger station, and then starts to climb the slope on the west. Switchbacks lead up to the base of the Redwall limestone in the lower end of Roaring Springs Canyon. There's no difficulty in locating the namesake spring—it's so loud it can be heard from the North Rim. At the head of Roaring Springs Canyon, the trail climbs steep switchbacks up to the rim and the North Kaibab Trailhead, 5.4 miles from Cottonwood Camp.

Tip: Since there is no water along the remainder of the route, go to the nearby North Rim Ranger Station to fill up on water for a dry camp later. Leave someone to watch your packs.

Continue the loop on the Ken Patrick Trail, which leaves the North Kaibab Trailhead and heads northwest across the Kaibab Plateau. Although the plateau is not level, the hiking is easy. Campsites, though dry, are plentiful in the gorgeous fir, spruce, and aspen forest. The Ken Patrick Trail crosses a tributary of Roaring Springs Canyon and the head of Bright Angel Creek before reaching the Cape Royal Road about a mile east of the Point Imperial Road junction. Follow the trail north along the rim of the canyon. This section of the Ken Patrick Trail has some great views of the head of Nankoweap Creek. The Ken Patrick Trail ends at the Point Imperial viewpoint, 7.5 miles from the North Kaibab Trailhead.

To finish the loop, hike northwest on an old fire road along the rim for 1.9 miles to the end of the Saddle Mountain Fire Road. Follow the Nankoweap Trail down the ridge to the west, toward Saddle Mountain. This upper section is little used now, and may be brushy. A 2.5-mile descent brings you to the saddle. Turn left on the Nankoweap Trail, hike north to the Saddle Mountain Trail, and turn left to return to the Saddle Mountain Trailhead.

	Camp	Miles	Elevation Gain
Day 1	Nankoweap Creek	7.4	1090
Day 2	Awatubi Creek	6.4	2940
Day 3	Mouth of Lava Canyon	7.1	720
Day 4	Unkar Creek	7.0	940
Day 5	Vishnu Creek	8.5	2840
Day 6	Clear Creek	8.7	890
Day 7	Bright Angel Campground	8.4	600
Day 8	Cottonwood Campground	6.8	1360
Day 9	North Rim	8.4	4560
Day 10	Out	10.0	890

SOUTH RIM VIA BRIGHT ANGEL TRAIL OPTIONAL FINISH If you left a vehicle at the Bright Angel Trailhead for the south rim exit, turn left from the Clear Creek–North Kaibab Trail junction, and hike 0.8 mile south on the North Kaibab Trail to Bright Angel Campground. Follow the River Trail from the Bright Angel Campground to the silver suspension bridge across the Colorado River, and west along the river to the mouth of Garden Creek and a stone rest house. Follow the Bright Angel Trail up Garden Canyon to Indian Gardens and on to the south rim and the Bright Angel Trailhead. Camping is allowed only at Indian Gardens Campground. You'll find piped water at Indian Gardens. During the summer you can get water at the two rest houses above Indian Gardens. It is 8.4 miles from the Clear Creek–North Kaibab Trail junction to Bright Angel Trailhead.

OPTIONAL SIDE HIKES From the Horse Thief Route, easy out-and-back side hikes are possible down lower Nankoweap and Kwagunt creeks to the Colorado River. You can also explore these canyons upstream from the Horse Thief Route. The descent of lower Malgosa Creek is more difficult than Kwagunt or Nankoweap creeks. Awatubi and 60 Mile creeks are not passable to the Colorado River. Unkar, Vishnu, and Clear creeks can be explored both up and downstream from the main route.

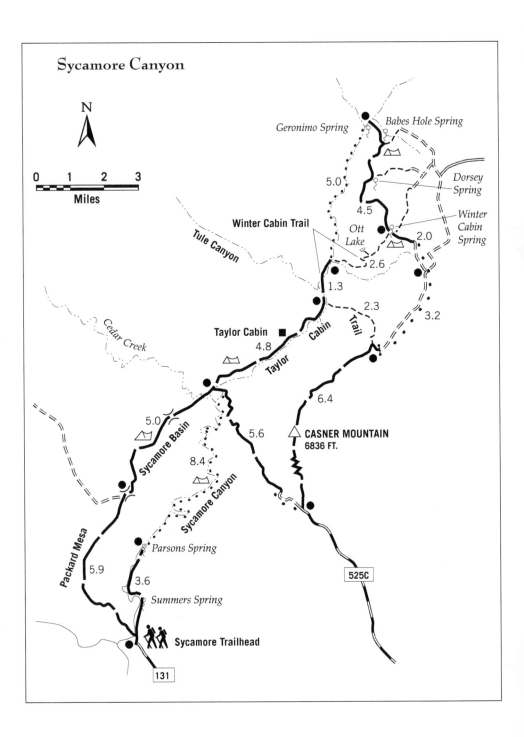

Sycamore Canyon

N

0 1 2 3
Miles

Geronimo Spring   Babes Hole Spring

5.0

4.5

Dorsey
Spring

Winter Cabin Trail

Ott
Lake

Winter
Cabin
Spring

2.0

2.6

Tule Canyon

1.3

2.3

3.2

Cedar Creek

Taylor Cabin

4.8

Cabin

Trail

Taylor

6.4

5.0

Sycamore Basin

5.6

CASNER MOUNTAIN
6836 FT.

8.4

Sycamore Canyon

Packard Mesa

Parsons Spring

5.9

3.6

Summers Spring

525C

Sycamore Trailhead

131

8 Sycamore Canyon

RATINGS (1–10)			MILES	ELEVATION GAIN	DAYS	SHUTTLE MILEAGE
Scenery	Solitude	Difficulty	55.7	6120	6	0
8	7	7				

MAPS Clarkdale, Sycamore Basin, Sycamore Point, Loy Butte U.S.G.S.

SEASON March–November.

BEST April–May, October–November.

WATER Lower Sycamore Creek to Parsons Spring, seasonal in upper Sycamore Creek, Geronimo Spring, Babes Hole Spring, Dorsey Spring, Winter Cabin Spring.

PERMITS A Red Rock Pass required for vehicle parking.

RULES Sycamore Canyon is closed to camping from Parsons Spring to the Verde River.

CONTACT Sedona Ranger District, Coconino National Forest, (928) 282-4119; Chino Valley Ranger District, Prescott National Forest, (928) 636-2302.

HIGHLIGHTS This is a long, rugged loop through a remote red rock canyon system. You will see few hikers on most of the hike. You'll start along a permanent creek, and loop up onto the Mogollon Rim through pine forest, before returning to the desert grasslands. Several optional trails can be used to make this a shorter loop, if desired.

PROBLEMS Sycamore Canyon drains a large area of the western Mogollon Rim, and often floods during the spring snow melt. From March through mid April, this trip may be impossible. On the other hand, after the snow melt ends, the creek rapidly dries up and you may have no water at all from Parsons Spring to Geronimo Spring, which is 20 miles of mostly cross-country hiking. You will need to carry water for overnight camps at least twice during this demanding loop.

HOW TO GET THERE From Cottonwood at the junction of Arizona 260 and Arizona 89A, drive 4 miles north on Main Street through downtown Cottonwood, toward Clarkdale. Turn right at the sign for Tuzigoot National Monument; drive 0.5 mile, crossing Verde River Bridge and turn left onto a maintained dirt road. Continue 10.3 miles to the end of the road at the Sycamore Trailhead.

Warning: Do not attempt this hike in the summer unless you are an experienced desert hiker. You'll find long stretches without water.

DESCRIPTION From the Sycamore Trailhead, start the hike on the Parsons Trail. This good trail immediately descends to Sycamore Creek and passes the junction with the Packard Mesa Trail, which is the return trail. Stay right and follow the Parsons Trail along the delightful perennial stream. After you pass Summers Spring, the trail becomes fainter as the canyon bends through a left-right S curve. Damage from the super floods of 1993 and 1994 is evident in the form of uprooted trees and piles of debris. At Parsons Spring, 3.6 miles from the trailhead, Sycamore Creek gradually emerges in a tangle of vegetation. Above this source, Sycamore Creek is normally dry, except during spring snowmelt or after a heavy summer thunderstorm. If the bed is dry, you will have to carry water for two dry camps. The next reliable water source is Geronimo Spring, 20 miles upstream from Parsons Spring.

Tip: If you time this trip well, just after the spring runoff but before the weather turns hot, there will still be deep, clear pools in Sycamore Creek, but not so much water that progress is difficult.

There is no trail upstream from Parsons Spring, so proceed by following the dry wash northeast. The canyon walls are composed of reddish sandstone layers of the Supai formation, which form an inner canyon about 400 feet deep. Luckily, the frequent floods keep the canyon bottom free of brush, so the cross-country walking is relatively easy. You'll probably want to camp along the canyon bottom somewhere east of Sycamore Basin.

At 12.0 miles from the Sycamore Trailhead, the cliffs forming the inner canyon taper away, and the Dogie Trail crosses Sycamore Creek to meet the Taylor Cabin and Sycamore Basin trails on the west bank. The Sycamore Basin Trail presents an option to shorten the loop.

To continue the main loop, turn right (northeast) on the Taylor Cabin Trail and follow this trail along the west side of Sycamore Creek. The trail is named for Taylor Cabin, an old rancher's line cabin recently restored by volunteers. The stone cabin is 2.8 miles from the trail junction, on the west bank of the creek. Upstream from the cabin the upper cliffs of Sycamore Canyon close in. Watch for the Taylor Cabin Trail turnoff 2.0 miles beyond the cabin. Here the Taylor Cabin Trail goes up an unnamed side canyon to the east, which offers another option for a shorter loop.

▲▲▲ Mogollon Rim

This 1000 to 2000-foot south-facing escarpment stretches 200 miles across central Arizona. The rim marks the division between the Colorado Plateau to the north, and the basin and range country to the south. The Colorado Plateau is characterized by layers of sedimentary rock cut by numerous canyons. In contrast, the basin and range country consists of parallel mountain ranges and intervening valleys.

Continue the main loop by hiking north on the obscure Winter Cabin Trail. The trail crosses the dry wash several times. If you lose the trail, just follow the bed of the wash upstream. Tule Canyon, a major side canyon, comes in from the left 0.7 mile upstream from the Taylor Cabin Trail. When you are 1.3 miles from the Taylor Cabin Trail, the Winter Cabin Trail exits Sycamore Canyon to the east, leaving the bed just north of an unnamed side canyon. The Winter Cabin Trail is the last option to make the loop shorter. This option is also useful if deep pools block the bed of Sycamore Canyon upstream of this point.

Warning: *Geronimo Spring is the only reliable water source in Sycamore Canyon above Parsons Spring.*

Hike cross-country up the dry bed of Sycamore Canyon to continue the main loop. There is a short but spectacular narrows in the buff Coconino sandstone about 2.5 miles from the Winter Cabin Trail. Little LO Spring Canyon comes in from the right (east) side of Sycamore Canyon, 5.0 miles from the Winter Cabin Trail. Walk 100

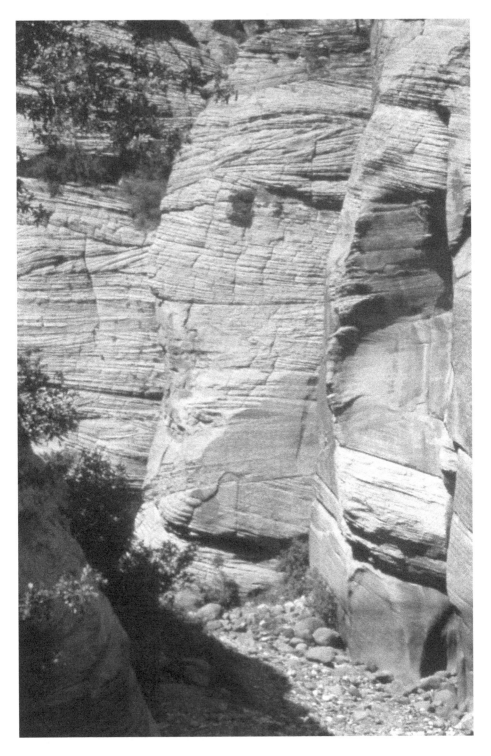

Coconino sandstone narrows, Sycamore Canyon

yards up this canyon to Geronimo Spring and the start of the Kelsey Trail.

Tip: An 0.2 mile side hike up Little LO Spring Canyon above Geronimo Spring reveals another spectacular narrows in the Coconino sandstone.

To continue the main loop, follow the Kelsey Trail as it climbs steeply out of Little LO Spring Canyon to the southeast. Just 0.5 mile of climbing brings you to Babes Hole Spring, where you'll turn right (south) on the Dorsey Trail. This trail follows an intermediate-level bench along the east side of Sycamore Canyon, and you'll pass through stands of ponderosa pine on the north-facing slopes. The trail levels off after another 1.5 miles and passes Dorsey Spring. Just 0.8 mile further on, the Dorsey Trail swings around a point onto a south-facing, brushy slope with great views south down Sycamore Canyon. After hiking 4.5 miles from Geronimo Spring, you'll reach Winter Cabin Spring, named for the ruins of an old log cabin.

Warning: Winter Cabin spring is the last reliable water on the return part of the loop. Plan to carry water for at least one, and probably two, dry camps.

Turn left (southeast) and follow the Winter Cabin Trail 1.4 miles to its end at the Winter Cabin Trailhead. Follow the trailhead road south 0.6 mile and turn right (southwest) on the Casner Mountain Road, which follows a high ridge. This forest road is used very little and it offers sweeping views of Sycamore Canyon on the west and Mooney Canyon on the east. After 3.0 miles, the road ends. Continue west on the Casner Mountain Trail 0.2 mile to an unnamed saddle and the Taylor Cabin Trail junction. The ridge narrows as you continue southwest on the Casner Mountain Trail. At the southwest end of the ridge, follow the trail over the mesa-like expanse of Casner Mountain. Descend the south side of the mountain along a series of switchbacks to the end of the trail at the Sycamore Pass Road, 6.4 miles southwest of the Taylor Cabin Trail. Turn right (northwest) and walk 1.4 miles to the Dogie Trailhead.

Continue on the Dogie Trail, which climbs over Sycamore Pass and heads northwest along the west slopes of Casner Mountain, which are dotted with small pinyon pines and junipers. The Dogie Trail stays on an intermediate terrace above Sycamore Canyon as it winds in and out of small drainages. You'll descend to cross

Sycamore Creek 4.2 miles from Sycamore Pass. Turn left and follow the Sycamore Basin Trail southwest across Cedar Creek.

Tip: In a pinch, you may be able to find water by walking cross-country a mile or two up Cedar Creek.

After crossing Cedar Creek, follow the Sycamore Basin Trail over an unnamed pass and down a gradual slope into Sycamore Basin. Sycamore Basin features good views of the upper rim of Sycamore Canyon to the west, and the inner canyon where you started the trip to the east. Easy walking brings you through another unnamed pass and the Sycamore Basin Trailhead, 5.0 miles from the Taylor Cabin Trail. Continue the main loop southwest on the Packard Mesa Trail. Easy walking though open grassland takes you 3.8 miles across the top of Packard Mesa to its southeast rim, where you'll descend 1.9 miles into Sycamore Creek. After crossing the creek, turn right on the Parsons Trail and go 0.2 mile south to the trailhead.

POSSIBLE ITINERARY

	Camp	Miles	Elevation Gain
Day 1	East of Sycamore Basin	8.2	390
Day 2	Taylor Cabin Trail turnoff	8.6	550
Day 3	Winter Cabin Spring	11.1	1940
Day 4	Dogie Trail	13.6	1790
Day 5	Sycamore Basin	7.5	930
Day 6	Out	6.7	520

SYCAMORE BASIN TRAIL OPTIONAL SHORTCUT From the junction of the Dogie, Taylor Cabin, and Sycamore Basin trails, turn left and return to the trailhead on the Sycamore Basin and Packard Mesa trails. This loop hike is a reasonable 2 to 3-day hike of 22.6 miles, with an elevation gain of 1260 feet.

TAYLOR CABIN TRAIL OPTIONAL SHORTCUT By leaving the main loop at the junction of the Taylor Cabin and Winter Cabin trails, you can do a loop of 41.8 miles, with 3220 feet of elevation gain—a good 4-day trek. Follow the Taylor Cabin Trail east up the unnamed drainage. Although the trail is rough and receives little maintenance, it is a gorgeous hike. As you climb, the mixed chaparral brush and pinyon-juniper give way to a forest of tall ponderosa pine and Douglas-fir. These evergreen conifers are growing on a north-facing slope well below their normal elevations. Follow the trail southeast up the steep slope. At about 2.0 miles from Sycamore Canyon the trail switchbacks to the right to gain the crest of a ridge. Your reward for the steep climb is great views down Sycamore Canyon. From this point, the trail runs east along the ridge and ends at the Casner Mountain Trail, 2.3 miles from Sycamore Canyon. Turn right and hike south on the Casner Mountain Trail to continue the main loop.

WINTER CABIN TRAIL OPTIONAL SHORTCUT Using the Winter Cabin Trail, you can shorten the loop to 48.7 miles with an elevation gain of 3200 feet. Allow 5 days for this hike. The unmarked Winter Cabin Trail leaves the bed of Sycamore Canyon just north of an unnamed side canyon. The Winter Cabin Trail is shown accurately on the U.S.G.S. topographic map, and you'll need the map to find the exit from Sycamore Canyon.

The trail is easy to follow, though little used. Follow it up the north side of the unnamed side canyon, and then into a tributary canyon. At the head of this drainage, follow the Winter Cabin Trail as it turns northwest, still climbing steadily. When the trail turns back to the east, watch for a 0.2-mile spur trail to Ott Lake. This little pond is usually dry, but the spot offers views of upper Sycamore Canyon. From the junction, continue the loop on the Winter Cabin Trail east through a saddle.

The trail levels off for the last mile to Winter Cabin Spring and the junction with the Dorsey Trail, 2.6 miles from and 1580 feet above Sycamore Creek. Turn right, remaining on the Winter Cabin Trail, to rejoin the main loop.

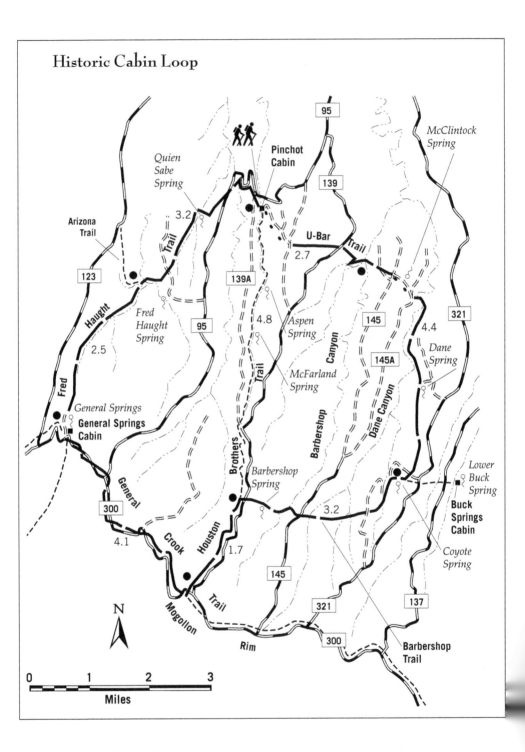

Historic Cabin Loop

Quien
Sabe
Spring

Pinchot
Cabin

McClintock
Spring

95

139

Arizona
Trail

3.2

Trail

U-Bar

Trail

2.7

123

Haught

95

139A

4.8

Aspen
Spring

145

321

4.4

Fred
Haught
Spring

McFarland
Spring

145A

Dane
Spring

2.5

Trail

Canyon

Fred

General Springs

General Springs
Cabin

Brothers

Barbershop
Spring

Barbershop

Dane Canyon

Lower
Buck
Spring

Buck
Springs
Cabin

General

300

Houston

3.2

4.1

Crook

1.7

145

Coyote
Spring

Mogollon

321

137

N

Trail

Rim

300

Barbershop
Trail

0   1   2   3
Miles

9 Historic Cabin Loop

RATINGS (1–10)			MILES	ELEVATION GAIN	DAYS	SHUTTLE MILEAGE
Scenery	Solitude	Difficulty	21.8	2860	3	0
7	6	4				

MAPS Blue Ridge Reservoir, Dane Canyon U.S.G.S.

SEASON April–November.

BEST April, October.

WATER Seasonal at Barbershop Canyon, McClintock Spring, Dane Canyon, Dane Spring, Coyote Spring, Lower Buck Spring, Barbershop Spring, General Springs, Fred Haught Spring, and Quien Sabe Spring. These water sources are reliable most years, but may go dry during droughts. Don't depend on any single source.

PERMITS None.

RULES None.

CONTACT Mogollon Rim District, Coconino National Forest, HC 31, Box 300, Happy Jack, Arizona 86024, (928) 477-2255, www.fs.fed.us/r3/coconino.

HIGHLIGHTS This relatively easy loop through magnificent ponderosa-pine forest follows historic trails and features historic cabins and hundred-mile views from the Mogollon Rim.

PROBLEMS This hike follows trails that parallel dirt roads at times. During hunting season, use caution and wear bright clothing.

HOW TO GET THERE From Flagstaff, drive 55 miles southeast on Lake Mary Road (Forest Highway 3) to the tiny hamlet of Clints Well. Turn left on Arizona Highway 87 and drive north 9 miles. Turn right (east) on Forest Road 95, a maintained dirt road. Follow this road 11.1 miles, turn left (south) on Forest Road 139A, and drive 0.1 mile to the

Fred Haught Trail crossing. Although signed, the trail crossing is not a formal trailhead, and parking is limited.

You can also reach Clints Well from Camp Verde and Interstate 17. Drive 30 miles east on the General Crook Trail (FH 9), turn left (north) on Arizona 87, and drive 11 miles to Clints Well.

DESCRIPTION This loop follows historic trails through the magnificent ponderosa pine, Douglas-fir, and quaking aspen forest of the Mogollon Rim country. These trails were used in the pioneer days to travel through this rugged country before modern highways and dirt roads were built. Most of these old trails have been lost to road construction or neglect. Recently, the U.S. Forest Service rediscovered the routes of several historic trails and restored them. However, some sections of the Cabin Loop receive little travel and may be faint. Although the Historic Cabin Loop is on the Coconino National Forest, the area is not a designated wilderness area. At times the trails parallel or cross dirt forest roads.

The Crossings

Travel in the country north of the Mogollon Rim is severely restricted by the network of canyons draining north from the rim into the Little Colorado River. Trails were built to take advantage of places where the canyons could be crossed, and many of these places were named. Some, such as Jones Crossing, are used by present-day forest roads. Others, such as Kinder Crossing and the unnamed crossings on the Cabin Loop, are still traversed by pack trails. Trail building was easy on the broad forested ridges, but required serious construction work in the canyons.

Follow the Fred Haught Trail east 0.2 mile to Pinchot Cabin, where it ends at the junction with the Houston Brothers and U-Bar trails. This cabin, 0.2 mile east of the trailhead, is the first of three historic cabins you'll pass on this hike. The U.S. Forest Service built the cabins as fire guard stations. In the days when this country was accessible primarily by trail, the Forest Service stationed fire crews and fire lookouts at numerous points throughout the forest. With the advent of helicopters and construction of more roads, the old cabins fell into disuse. Recently, the Forest Service restored the three cabins on this loop hike. Pinchot Cabin is named for Gifford Pinchot, the first Chief of the Forest Service, who visited this idyllic spot during his tenure.

Walk past the cabin and start up the U-Bar Trail, which follows an old road east out of the shallow canyon. This section of the U-Bar Trail is the most confusing because the trail follows two-track roads as well as a faint trail tread. Follow the tree blazes carefully. Be especially alert for the places where the trail leaves a road.

Warning: Pay close attention to tree blazes to avoid losing the trail, especially on the flat ridge tops. If you do lose it, backtrack to the last known blaze, and look for the trail from there.

The entire trail has been marked with fresh blazes, and the tread is becoming more distinct as the old trail receives more use. Also, look for old, historic blazes dating from the original construction of the trail.

After following roads for 1.0 mile, the U-Bar Trail heads east to cross Dick Hart Draw. On the far side of the shallow draw, follow the trail across a broad ridge and Forest Road 139, a maintained dirt road. East of the road, the U-Bar Trail descends into Barbershop Canyon, where you'll see some of the original trail construction. The trail crosses Barbershop Canyon at the confluence of Merritt Draw, 2.5 miles from Pinchot Cabin. You'll probably find seasonal water in Barbershop Canyon.

After the U-Bar Trail climbs out of Barbershop Canyon, it crosses a road, joins another road, and passes by McClintock Spring. Watch carefully for the point where the trail leaves the road and descends into Dane Canyon, 3.7 miles from Pinchot Cabin. You'll find several small campsites and seasonal water in Dane Canyon.

Tip: The best campsites are on the ridges, though you'll have to carry water for a dry camp.

On the east side of Dane Canyon, follow the U-Bar Trail as it turns south and parallels Dane Canyon as it heads toward Dane Spring.

From Dane Spring, follow the U-Bar Trail south up an unnamed draw. Cross a broad ridge and descend into an unnamed drainage, where the U-Bar Trail ends at the junction with the Barbershop Trail, 6.9 miles from Pinchot Cabin. As an option, you can turn left on the Barbershop Trail and visit Buck Springs Cabin, the second of the historic cabins on the Cabin Loop.

☀ Montane Ponderosa Pine Forest

This forest community is the primary forest type in Arizona, covering much of the high country between about 6000 and 8000 feet. Also known as the transition zone because of C. Hart Merriam's lifezone work, these forests are almost pure stands of ponderosa pine. Ponderosa pines are found in every western state, but only in Arizona are conditions right for a vast, pure ponderosa forest. Gambel oak, a slender deciduous tree about 20 to 30 feet high, grows in the ponderosa forest, favoring rocky outcrops. Another forest resident, the tassle-eared or Abert's squirrel, flirts its long fluffy tail at hikers as it scampers easily from branch to branch, high in the tree crowns. You may also hear the harsh call of the Steller's jay, a large blue jay with a crested head. Flocks of tiny pygmy nuthatches roam the forest, settling in the tree crowns and working their way down the tree, inverted, looking for tasty insects in the bark.

From the junction of the U-Bar and Barbershop Trails, continue the loop by turning right (west) and following the Barbershop Trail down the unnamed drainage. Coyote Spring is along this drainage. The trail soon meets a road and follows it south into Bill Mc-Clintock Draw. Watch carefully for the point where the Barbershop Trail leaves the road in a meadow and heads west as a foot trail. The Barbershop Trail crosses three broad ridges before descending into upper Dane Canyon, where you may find seasonal water. Continue west on the Barbershop Trail across Forest Road 145, a maintained dirt road, and down into upper Barbershop Canyon. Look carefully for the trail leaving the canyon to the west. It passes Barbershop Spring before climbing to cross Forest Road 139 on a broad ridge. Just 0.1 mile beyond the road, the Barbershop Trail ends at the junction with the Houston Brothers Trail, 3.2 miles from the end of the U-Bar

𝕁 General Crook Trail

General George Crook built this wagon road during the Apache Indian Wars as a supply route connecting several U.S. Army forts in central Arizona. The present-day trail, marked by white chevrons nailed to trees, follows the original route. The wagon road is still visible in many places. The modern Rim Road (Forest Road 300) closely parallels the General Crook Trail.

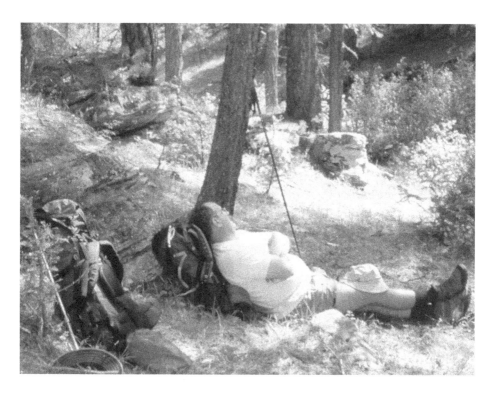

Lunch stop, Barbershop Canyon, U-Bar Trail

🔥 Dude Fire

Views from the Mogollon Rim are excellent, but unfortunately they are somewhat marred by the dead forest left in the aftermath of the Dude Fire. This huge fire started south of the rim in 1990 and burned large tracts of the Tonto National Forest before being stopped along the Mogollon Rim, which marks the boundary of the Coconino National Forest. Large, destructive forest fires occur with increasing frequency in the American Southwest. Under presettlement conditions, low intensity fires swept through the ponderosa forests every few years, thinning the underbrush and creating an open, parklike forest. A century of aggressive fire suppression, heavy grazing, and poor timber harvest methods have left much of Arizona's forests crowded with small pines. Such "doghair" stands burn hot, and the resulting fire often gets into the tree tops, resulting in destructive crown fires. One management response is to set "prescribed fires," under carefully controlled conditions, in roaded areas such as the Cabin Loop area. These fires mimic the actions of natural fires, reducing the fuel load and the intensity of future wild fires.

Trail. An optional shortcut uses the Houston Brothers Trail to return to the trailhead near Pinchot Cabin.

To continue the main loop, turn left (south) and follow the Houston Brothers Trail as it loosely parallels Forest Road 139 just to the west. This trail was named for two pioneer ranching brothers in the rim country. The Houston Brothers Trail heads several small canyons as it works its way south. You'll cross Forest Road 300 and reach the junction with the General Crook Trail at the Mogollon Rim, 1.7 miles from the end of the Barbershop Trail.

Turn right and follow the General Crook Trail, which is marked with white chevrons nailed to trees. The Rim Road, Forest Road 300, is always nearby, and the old trail crosses the modern road several times.

Tip: *At several points, you can get sweeping views from the edge of the Mogollon Rim by walking a few yards south from the trail.*

Stay on the General Crook Trail 4.1 miles, and then turn right on the signed spur road to General Springs Cabin. Walk north 0.3 mile down this road to General Springs Cabin, the third historic cabin on the loop. General Springs normally has water, and there is seasonal water along General Springs Canyon to the north. At the cabin, go north on the Fred Haught Trail, which follows General Springs Canyon. This is also the route of the Arizona Trail. In the spring, you'll pass several small cascades along the upper section of General Springs Canyon. The canyon becomes deeper as it gradually turns northeast.

Arizona Trail

Conceived by Flagstaff schoolteacher Dale Shewalter, this ambitious 800-mile trail traverses the scenic heart of Arizona from the Utah to Mexican borders. It uses existing trails such as the Fred Haught Trail, as well as old roads and new trail construction.

When you've walked 2.5 miles from General Springs Cabin, the Arizona Trail forks left and leaves General Springs Canyon. Stay right on the Fred Haught Trail, which continues just a few yards down General Springs Canyon before turning right up Fred Haught Canyon. Just 0.3 mile from the Arizona Trail junction, the trail passes a short spur trail to Fred Haught Spring, turns left (north), and climbs over a saddle. After crossing a road, the trail drops into the head of Quien Sabe Draw, which it follows downstream to the north. After you pass Quien Sabe Spring, follow the Fred Haught Trail right up a draw, cross Forest Road 95 on the ridge top, and descend to briefly follow Forest Road 95 across Bear Canyon. After 0.2 mile, the trail leaves the road on the right, and climbs up to the crossing on Forest Road 139A, your starting point.

POSSIBLE ITINERARY

	Camp	Miles	Elevation Gain
Day 1	Coyote Spring	6.9	1460
Day 2	General Springs	9.0	920
Day 3	Out	5.9	480

BUCK SPRINGS CABIN OPTIONAL SIDE HIKE From the junction of the U-Bar and Barbershop Trails, turn left (east) on the Barbershop Trail and walk 0.75 mile to the Barbershop Trailhead and Buck Springs Cabin, the second of the historic cabins on the Cabin Loop. Lower Buck Springs is about 0.2 mile northeast of the cabin.

HOUSTON BROTHERS TRAIL OPTIONAL SHORTCUT From the junction of the Barbershop and Houston Brothers trails, turn right (north) and follow the Houston Brothers Trail 4.8 miles back to Pinchot Cabin. With this option, the loop is 14.9 miles and can be done as a 2-day trip. The trail parallels Forest Road 139 just to the west, working its way through the heads of several side canyons, before crossing Forest Road 139A and descending gradually into the head of Houston Draw. The Houston Brothers Trail wanders through delightful aspen-lined meadows and passes several springs enroute to Pinchot Cabin. At the cabin, turn left (west) on the Fred Haught Trail and walk 0.2 mile to Forest Road 139A, your starting point.

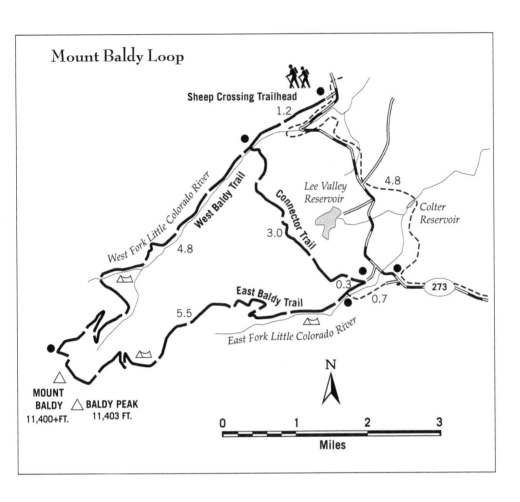

Mount Baldy Loop

Sheep Crossing Trailhead
1.2

West Fork Little Colorado River

West Baldy Trail

Connector Trail

Lee Valley Reservoir

4.8

Colter Reservoir

4.8

3.0

0.3

0.7

273

East Baldy Trail

5.5

East Fork Little Colorado River

N

MOUNT
BALDY △ BALDY PEAK
11,400+FT.   11,403 FT.

0   1   2   3
Miles

10 Mount Baldy Loop

RATINGS (1–10)			MILES	ELEVATION GAIN	DAYS	SHUTTLE MILEAGE
Scenery	Solitude	Difficulty	15.8	2760	2	0
9	5	6	(16.8)	(2800)	(2)	

MAPS Mount Baldy, Big Lake North U.S.G.S.

SEASON June–November.

BEST July–October.

WATER West Fork Little Colorado River, East Fork Little Colorado River.

PERMITS None.

RULES None.

CONTACT Springerville Ranger District, Apache-Sitgreaves National Forest, P.O. Box 760 Springerville, Arizona 85938, (928) 333-4372, www.fs.fed.us/r3/asnf.

HIGHLIGHTS This is a scenic hike along two trout streams and the summit of Arizona's second highest mountain.

PROBLEMS The east boundary of the White Mountain Apache Reservation runs along the summit ridge of Mount Baldy. The reservation is permanently closed to all entry, and violators have been fined and had their equipment confiscated. Baldy Peak, the highest named summit, is within the reservation and is off limits to hikers. However, the actual high point of the mountain is a point along the ridge 0.4 mile to the north. This point is within the national forest and is open to hikers.

HOW TO GET THERE From Springerville, drive 3 miles south on U.S. 180 to Eagar and turn right on Arizona 260. Continue west 16 miles; turn left on Arizona 273 and drive 8.7 miles to the Sheep Crossing Trailhead, on the right. This paved highway becomes all-weather gravel when you enter the national forest. The lush alpine meadows on this hike have long been used to graze sheep during the summer, which is the origin of the name "Sheep Crossing." The crossing is the only convenient point to cross the West Fork, which briefly emerges from its high mountain canyon only to drop into another deep canyon immediately downstream.

DESCRIPTION-This delightful loop in Arizona's White Mountains is made possible by a couple of new trails that connect the West and East Baldy Trailheads. The Connector Trail is not shown on the topographic maps, and the West and East Baldy Trails are shown incorrectly. From Sheep Crossing Trailhead, follow the West Baldy Trail southwest through gently sloping, open forest. After 1.2 miles the trail descends into a valley and follows the West Fork of the Little Colorado River upstream to the southwest. The West Fork is more of a creek than a river high in the headwaters.

～～ Headwaters of the Little Colorado River

The Little Colorado River rises near the summit of Mount Baldy. Both the East and West Forks are small mountain creeks. After the two forks join, northeast of the Sheep Crossing Trailhead, the river continues to the north and northwest, eventually joining the Colorado River in the Grand Canyon.

Turn left (southeast) on the Connector Trail 1.4 miles from the Sheep Crossing Trailhead. Cross the West Fork on a couple of logs and follow the Connector Trail as it climbs steadily up a ridge to the south, passing through dense, gorgeous alpine forest of Douglas-fir, Colorado blue spruce, and quaking aspen. After 1.0 mile, you'll pass through a saddle, where the trail swings southeast and drops into a small meadow at the head of a tributary canyon. The trail climbs over another ridge and passes through a second meadow before wandering through the trees to reach a third meadow, which is the largest along the Connector Trail. At the southeast corner of this meadow, the trail enters the forest and descends southeast to the East Baldy Trailhead, 3.0 miles from the West Baldy and Connector Trail junction. At the East Baldy Trailhead, turn right on the East Baldy Trail,

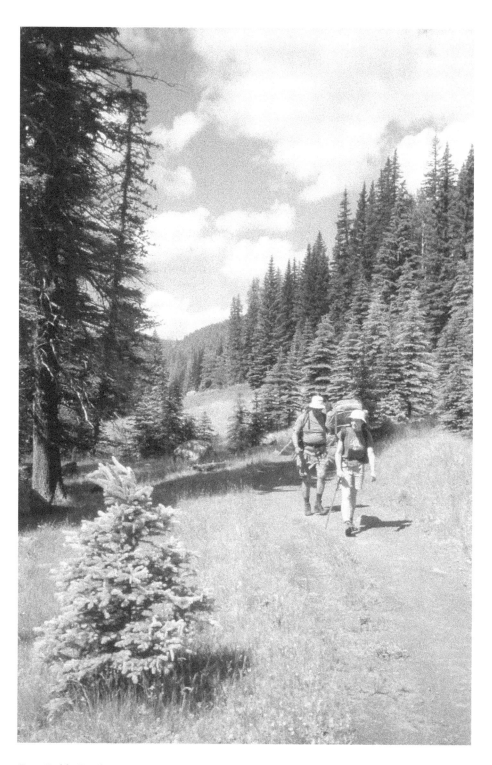

East Baldy Trail, Mount Baldy Wilderness

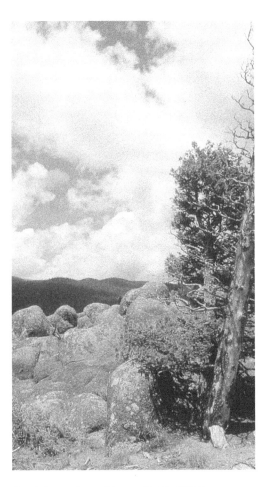
Rock formations, Mount Baldy Wilderness

which heads southwest up the East Fork of the Little Colorado River.

After you've hiked 0.3 mile, the trail descends to the East Fork and a side trail from the Gabaldon Horse Campground comes in from the left. Stay right, on the north side of the creek, and follow the East Baldy Trail out of the forest into a broad meadow. You'll find numerous campsites across the creek, along the south side of this unnamed meadow.

Tip: *It is 6.7 miles to the West Fork, the next reliable water source.*

Just after entering the meadow, bear right at an unsigned fork in the trail. Follow the East Baldy Trail as it climbs gradually up the north slope of the valley and goes in and out of small meadows. Eventually, the trail climbs through a series of cliffs and pinnacles, and switchbacks to the top of the unnamed ridge north of the East Fork. You'll find several good campsites along this ridge, but you'll need to carry water from the East Fork for a dry camp.

Warning: *From this point until the trail drops into the West Fork, you'll be hiking along high, exposed ridges. From July through mid-September, afternoon thunderstorms are common in the mountains. Plan your hike to be off the ridges by noon.*

The trail passes along the top of several rock outcrops and provides views of the bald summit ridge of Mount Baldy to the west and of the White Mountains to the south and east. After this open

♈ Mount Baldy: Views and Subalpine Forest

From the summit of Mount Baldy, much of eastern Arizona is visible. The sprawling mass of the White Mountains lies at your feet. These volcanic mountains were built up from a series of lava flows and cinder cone eruptions. This is the reason the range is loftier than the Mogollon Rim country to the west and east. On a clear day, you can see the San Francisco Mountains, Arizona's highest mountains, 150 miles to the northwest. To the east and southeast, closer at hand, lie the rugged and remote Blue Range Primitive Area along the eastern border of the state, and the rounded summits of the Mogollon Mountains, in the Gila Wilderness in New Mexico. Mount Baldy is the headwaters for the Little Colorado, the Black, and the White rivers, all of which eventually flow into the master river of the Southwest, the Colorado.

Mount Baldy is crowned with a beautiful forest dominated by Englemann spruce and corkbark fir. With their spire-like crowns, these trees are adapted to the heavy snow that falls at elevations above 10,000 feet. Although the top of Mount Baldy receives around 40 inches of precipitation per year, much of it as snow, the summer monsoon also contributes significant moisture.

The lower limit of the subalpine spruce-fir forest is marked by the transition to a mixed forest of quaking aspen, Douglas-fir, white fir, and blue spruce. The upper limit is marked by timberline, which is just barely reached on the summit ridge of Mount Baldy.

Above timberline, weather conditions are too harsh for trees to survive. At timberline, the struggle for life creates interesting interactions between forest and tundra. Trees grow in tree islands, bunched together against the icy wind. Individual trees hunker down behind boulders that block the prevailing wind, and are sculpted into fantastic shapes as the shrub-like tree fills all the of the protected space. Limbs that attempt to grow beyond the shelter of the island or boulder are promptly frost nipped and die back. Such bizarrely shaped trees are called "krummholtz."

A distinctive bird found in this high-altitude forest is the Clark's nutcracker. A large gray, white, and black jay, the Clark's nutcracker is also known as the "camp robber" because of its tendency to raid campsites for tidbits.

section, the trail enters the forest once again and works its way west along the ridge. As you gain elevation, the mixed forest of quaking aspen and Douglas-fir gives way to a beautiful mixture of subalpine and Arizona corkbark fir. The trail ends 5.8 miles from the East Baldy Trailhead, at the start of the West Baldy Trail on the north ridge of Mount Baldy, just below timberline.

Tip: To reach the highest point of Mount Baldy, hike 0.4 mile south on an unmaintained trail to the highest point of the summit ridge. This high point is near the letter "O" in the label "MOUNT BALDY" on the topographic map.

This high point is at least 11,400 feet, the elevation of the highest contour line on the topographic map. It's likely that this high point is a few feet higher than 11,403-foot Baldy Peak, which is visible 0.4 miles further south.

To continue the main loop, follow the West Baldy Trail north as it descends along the northeast ridge of Mount Baldy. The trail descends into the headwaters of the West Fork via a long switchback. After this switchback, the West Baldy Trail turns northeast, then northwest around the end of the ridge and crosses a tributary of the West Fork, 2.0 miles from the East and West Baldy Trail junction.

Warning: Do not attempt to hike south along the ridge to Baldy Peak, which is in the White Mountain Apache Reservation. Apache rangers patrol the summit area (there is a logging road just below Baldy Peak on the reservation side), and hikers have been arrested and fined for illegally entering the reservation. The reservation boundary runs along the west side of the "Mount Baldy" summit ridge, and is marked on the ground by low metal posts. At the south end of the summit ridge, the boundary turns east, putting Baldy Peak inside the reservation and off limits.

Follow the West Baldy Trail along the valley bottom near the creek. The trail passes through several meadows, and you'll find plenty of campsites.

Tip: Place your camp as far from the stream as possible, and out of sight of the trail. This is a very popular trail, and keeping your camp out of sight increases the wilderness experience for you and other hikers.

You'll reach the Connector Trail junction 4.8 miles from the East and West Baldy Trail junction, closing the loop. Continue another 1.2 miles on the West Baldy Trail to reach the Sheep Crossing Trailhead.

	Camp	Miles	Elevation Gain
Day 1	East Fork	5.0	730
Day 2	Out	10.8	2030

APACHE RAILROAD TRAIL OPTION The Apache Railroad Trail, the route of a former scenic railroad, offers a scenic alternative to the Connector Trail. From the east end of the Sheep Crossing Trailhead parking area, descend a few yards south to the Apache Railroad Trail and turn right. Follow the old railroad grade southwest along the West Fork just above Arizona 273. The highway soon crosses the West Fork, but the trail continues a little further upstream before crossing. After crossing the West Fork, the Apache Railroad Trail turns east and crosses the gravel highway 1.2 miles from the Sheep Crossing Trailhead. Follow the trail around the end of a ridge. The Apache Railroad Trail crosses the side road to Winn Campground 2.7 miles from the Sheep Crossing Trailhead and swings away from the gravel highway, looping east across an expansive meadow. It crosses the earthen dam that forms tiny Colter Reservoir, parallels the tree line, and heads south. This entire section offers views of the mass of Mount Baldy to the west. At 4.7 miles, the trail parallels Arizona 273 again. Leave the trail here, cross the road, and walk west 0.3 mile up the side road to Gabaldon Horse Campground. At the west end of the campground, start up the East Baldy Trail, follow it 0.5 mile to the junction with the hiker's East Baldy Trail, and turn left (west) to join the loop hike over Mount Baldy.

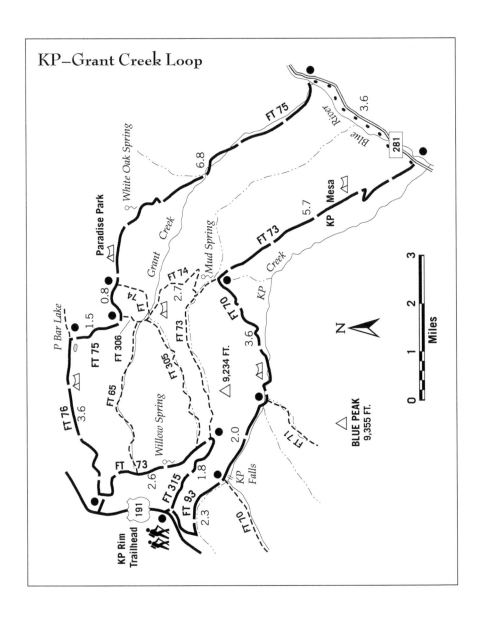

KP–Grant Creek Loop

FT 75

Blue River

3.6

281

White Oak Spring

6.8

Paradise Park

Grant Creek

Mud Spring

KP Mesa

FT 73

5.7

KP Creek

P Bar Lake

0.8

FT 74

FT 74

2.7

1.5

FT 75

FT 306

FT 73

FT 70

3.6

9,234 FT.

N

FT 65

FT 305

Willow Spring

0 1 2 3

Miles

FT 76

3.6

BLUE PEAK
9,355 FT.

FT 71

FT 73

2.6

FT 315

1.8

2.0

KP
Falls

191

FT 93

2.3

FT 70

KP Rim
Trailhead

11   KP--Grant Creek Loop

RATINGS (1–10)			MILES	ELEVATION GAIN	DAYS	SHUTTLE MILEAGE
Scenery	Solitude	Difficulty	34.6	4440	4	0
7	7	6	(21.1)	(2830)	(2–3)	

MAPS Strayhorse, Bear Mountain, Beaverhead, Hannagan Meadow U.S.G.S., Blue Range Primitive and Wilderness Areas U.S.F.S.

SEASON May–November.

BEST June–October.

WATER KP Creek, Blue River, Grant Creek, White Oak Spring, Willow Spring.

PERMITS None.

RULES None.

CONTACT Alpine Ranger District, Apache-Sitgreaves National Forest, P.O. Box 469 Alpine, Arizona 85920, (928) 339-4384, www.fs.fed.us/r3/asnf.

HIGHLIGHTS This loop trip features a wide variety of seldom-visited trails in the western section of the Blue Range Primitive Area. The hike starts from the dense fir-aspen forest along the KP Rim, and loops down to the Blue River in semi-desert juniper forest, before climbing back to the KP Rim via a scenic canyon.

PROBLEMS Lingering snowdrifts may block the trail along the western high-elevation section of the trip until June. In the fall, the first winter storms normally occur in November, but can start as early as October. Although hiking through the tapestry of fall colors during October is a treat, keep a wary eye on the weather. On the other hand, the lower sections of this route along the Blue River are hot during June and July.

HOW TO GET THERE From Alpine, drive 24 miles south on U.S. 191; turn left into the KP Rim Trailhead parking area.

DESCRIPTION From the KP Rim Trailhead, start the hike on Forest Trail 93. (Forest Trail 315 also leaves this trailhead, and is the return route.) Forest Trail 93 descends south through magnificent fir and aspen forest into an unnamed tributary of KP Creek. (The U.S. Forest Service uses numbers rather than names to refer to Blue Range trails on signs and maps, so I've done likewise.) When the trail reaches the bottom of the unnamed canyon, it turns east and follows the drainage downstream. Forest Trail 93 ends at Forest Trail 70, 2.3 miles from the trailhead, where the KP Creek Trail and KP Creek come in from the right. Stay left on the KP Creek trail and follow it east down perennial KP Creek. KP Falls, a small, pretty cascade, is on the right just beyond the trail junction. As you continue downstream there are a few small campsites along the creek.

> *Tip:* If you use one of these campsites, be extra careful with camp sanitation. Broadcast dish water at least 100 yards from the creek, and answer the call of nature at least 300 yards from water to avoid polluting this pristine mountain stream.

The KP Creek Trail drops into the creek bed and crosses it several times. This section is a bit slow, as floods have washed out the trail. Forest Trail 71 joins from the left 2.0 miles from KP Falls. Follow the KP Creek Trail along the creek for another mile.

> *Tip:* When the trail starts to climb away from the creek to the northeast, pick up water for a dry camp. There are no permanent water sources until you reach the Blue River, 8 miles away.

As the trail leaves the moist, sheltered canyon floor, the vegetation changes to pinyon pine and juniper forest, with a few stands of

⚘ Montane Mixed-Conifer Forest

The rim along the northwest boundary of the Blue Range is covered with a delightful mix of Douglas-fir, white fir, blue spruce, and quaking aspen. Because of the abundant moisture from deep winter snow and heavy summer rains, this mountain forest is one of the most diverse in the state—and certainly one of the prettiest. The forest is home to black bear, mule deer, wild turkey, and elk.

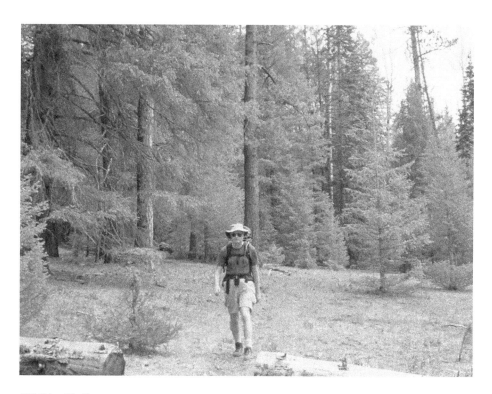

KP Rim Trail

ponderosa pine. Forest Trail 70 ends after another 2.6 miles, at the junction with Forest Trail 73.

> **Tip:** *Mud Spring, a seasonal water source, is located about 0.3 mile to the left, in the bed of Steeple Creek.*

From this junction, the optional Moonshine Park shortcut makes the trip a day or two shorter.

Continue the main loop south of Mud Spring by turning right (southeast) on Forest Trail 73. The trail follows a long ridge that eventually leads out onto Steeple and KP mesas, overlooking the deep canyon carved out by KP Creek. Both mesas offer unlimited camping in open pinyon pine and juniper forest, but you'll have to carry water from KP Creek or Mud Spring. At the southeast end of KP Mesa, the trail switchbacks off the rim and starts a steep descent to end at the Blue Road, Forest Road 281, about 5.7 miles from Forest Trail 70.

Turn left and hike north 3.6 miles on Forest Road 281; turn left (northwest) on Forest Trail 75. You may find seasonal water along the lower section of the creek, and there are a few campsites. Forest Trail

Backpackers in the Blue Range have the exciting possibility of seeing or hearing a wolf. In 1998, Mexican Gray Wolves were reintroduced in the Apache National Forest as part of a program to rescue the wolves from the edge of extinction. Only about 200 Mexican Gray Wolves survive, most in captive breeding programs. Currently, about two dozen wolves range freely in the wolf recovery area, which includes the Gila National Forest in New Mexico and the Apache National Forest (including the Blue Range) in Arizona

75 climbs gradually along the creek for 3.2 miles, then leaves the bed and climbs out of the canyon along a ridge. This steep climb takes you past seasonal White Oak Spring. The trail turns more westerly as it heads into Paradise Park. In the Blue Range, the term "park" usually refers to a meadow, but Paradise Park is more a ponderosa-pine flat than a meadow. Still, it's a pleasant change from the steep climb you just finished, as the trail wanders through the majestic pines. Forest Trail 74 comes in from the left, 6.8 miles from the Blue River. Continue straight (west) on Forest Trail 75, and watch for another trail on the left, Forest Trail 306, which joins after 0.8 mile. This is the point where the Moonshine Park optional short-cut joins the main loop. Stay right on Forest Trail 75 as it starts climbing and crosses an unnamed creek below an unnamed spring.

Tip: This creek is the last water source for the next 6.5 miles of the route. If the creek is dry, you may want to retrace your steps, and follow Forest Trail 306 for 0.4 mile to Grant Creek for water and campsites.

After crossing the creek, follow a single switchback on the west side of the unnamed canyon to a viewpoint overlooking the western Blue Range. After the switchback, the trail climbs steadily to P Bar Lake, a muddy, seasonal pond at the junction with Forest Trail 76.

Turn left (west) on Forest Trail 76 and follow the nearly level trail as it wanders through the fir and aspen forest. There's unlimited camping, but no water except for the unpalatable-looking stuff in P Bar Lake. In late spring, though, you'll probably encounter snowdrifts that you can melt for water. Forest Trail 76 continues west to end at the Hannagan Meadow Trailhead, near U.S. 191. Turn left onto Forest Trail 73, and follow this trail down a shallow drainage, a tributary of Grant Creek. You'll find plenty of campsites as the trail passes through meadows and climbs over low, forested saddles. Seasonal water flows in the small creeks. You'll soon pass the west end of Forest Trail 65 at the head of Grant Creek. Continue straight (south) on Forest Trail 73 past Willow Spring, set in a gorgeous alpine meadow. South of this spring, you'll also pass the west end of Forest Trail 305 and meet Forest Trail 315 on the north rim of KP Creek canyon. Turn sharply right (west) and follow the trail west along the edge of the 1700-foot-deep gorge. Just 1.8 miles of easy walking take you to the KP Rim Trailhead and the end of the loop.

POSSIBLE ITINERARY

	Camp	Miles	Elevation Gain
Day 1	Mud Spring	7.9	400
Day 2	Lower Grant Creek	9.9	400
Day 3	P Bar Lake	8.6	3300
Day 4	Out	8.2	340

MOONSHINE PARK OPTIONAL SHORTCUT From the junction of Forest Trails 73 and 70, turn left (north) onto Forest Trail 73, and hike 0.6 mile past Mud Spring to Forest Trail 74. Turn right (east) and follow this trail out of the Steeple Creek canyon, around a ridge, and north past Moonshine Park.

Tip: The U.S.G.S. topographic map incorrectly shows the trail passing west of Moonshine Park. Actually, the trail passes along the rim of Grant Creek, several hundred yards to the east. A spur trail leads to the park, which is not visible from the main trail.

The ponderosa-pine forest around this small meadow offers almost unlimited camping. The nearest water is Steeple Creek and Mud Spring to the south, or Grant Creek, about a mile north. Continue northwest on Forest Trail 74 and contour into Grant Creek. You'll find campsites here, and Grant Creek normally has water. Just after you reach the creek, you'll reach the junction with Forest Trail 65. Turn left on Forest Trail 65 and continue up Grant Creek. Just 0.1 mile further, Forest Trail 305 branches left. Stay right (west) on Forest Trail 65 along Grant Creek. After 0.2 mile, turn right (north) on Forest Trail 306. Follow the trail as it climbs out of Grant Creek to meet Forest Trail 75. Turn left on Forest Trail 75 to rejoin the main loop.

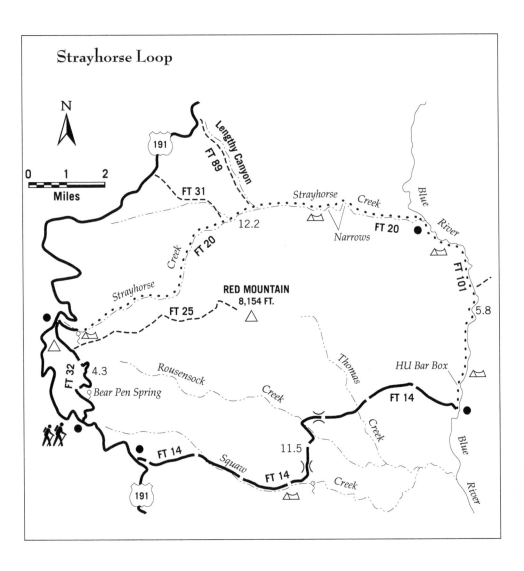

Strayhorse Loop

N

0 1 2
Miles

191

Lengthy Canyon

FT 89

FT 31

Strayhorse Creek

12.2

Narrows

FT 20

Blue River

FT 20

FT 101

Strayhorse Creek

RED MOUNTAIN
8,154 FT.

FT 25

5.8

FT 32

4.3

Rousensock

Thomas

HU Bar Box

Bear Pen Spring

Creek

Creek

FT 14

11.5

FT 14

Squaw

FT 14

Creek

Blue River

191

12 Strayhorse Loop

RATINGS (1–10)			MILES	ELEVATION GAIN	DAYS	SHUTTLE MILEAGE
Scenery	Solitude	Difficulty	33.8	4240	5	2.3
7	9	7				(see text)

MAPS Rose Peak, Dutch Blue Creek U.S.G.S., Blue Range Primitive and Wilderness Areas U.S.F.S.

SEASON May–November.

BEST September–October.

WATER Strayhorse Spring, Strayhorse Creek, Blue River, Rousensock Creek, and Squaw Creek.

PERMITS None.

RULES None.

CONTACT Alpine Ranger District, Apache-Sitgreaves National Forest, P.O. Box 469 Alpine, Arizona 85920, (928) 339-4384; Clifton Ranger District, Apache-Sitgreaves National Forest, HC 1, Box 733, Duncan, Arizona 85534, (520) 687-1301, www.fs.fed.us/r3/asnf.

HIGHLIGHTS This loop takes you through the remote southwest corner of the Blue Range Primitive Area and includes a unique section of hiking along the Blue River. You are unlikely to see any other people on this hike. In fact, it has the flavor of hiking in Arizona before the recreation explosion, when trailheads were rarely marked, back-country trails were almost unused, and trail signs often missing.

PROBLEMS This is a demanding hike due to the condition of the trails. Although the Forest Service wilderness map shows this entire loop as following system trails, the trails receive little maintenance. The trail down Strayhorse Canyon is now mostly a blazed route and should be considered cross-country, although there are occasional sections of good trail.

Tip: *If this loop is hiked clockwise, as described, you'll encounter the roughest hiking near the start of the loop, rather than at the end when you are committed to finishing it.*

Periodic floods on the Blue River have removed nearly all trace of the Blue River Trail, although there was probably never an actual constructed trail along the flood plain, just a path beaten in by horsemen.

Warning: *During spring snowmelt, the western portion of the loop may be blocked by deep snow, and the creeks may be running too high for passage, especially Strayhorse Creek. The Blue River portion of the loop requires frequent fording of the Blue River, which will be difficult and possibly dangerous during the runoff.*

HOW TO GET THERE From Alpine, drive 50.3 miles south on U.S. 191 to Forest Trail 32 at Hogtrail Saddle. This is the starting point, but since the exit trailhead is just 2.3 miles further south on the highway, you might want to leave your packs here, along with most of the group, and have someone park at the Squaw Creek Trailhead (Forest Trail 14) and walk back to Hogtrail Saddle on the highway.

Tip: *This trip is best hiked in the fall, after the summer monsoon ends (approximately mid-September), when the creeks and the Blue River are low. You'll also be treated to fall color, either in the riparian forest along the Blue River, or in the alpine fir-aspen forest at the start and end of the loop.*

DESCRIPTION The hike starts on the Bear Pen Trail (Forest Trail 32), which gradually climbs north along the east side of Rose Peak and its satellite ridges. Because of the southern exposure, the slopes are covered with a mixture of chaparral brush, junipers, and pinyon pines. The excellent view to the east encompasses all of the country you'll traverse on the loop. After 1.5 miles, an unsigned, blazed trail leads down a side canyon about 0.1 mile to Bear Pen Spring, which usually has a small but usable flow. After the trail turns northwest below Rose Peak itself, the slopes become forested with pine, fir, and aspen. Soon, you'll pass the Red Mountain Trail, which joins from the right. Another mile of pleasant hiking brings you to the Rose Peak Trailhead.

Continue east on the Strayhorse Creek Trail (Forest Trail 20), which starts from the unsigned trailhead at the backcountry infor-

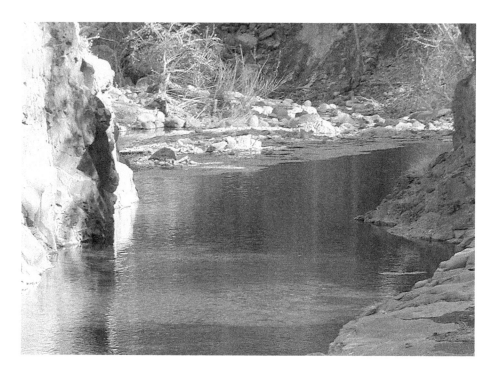

Strayhorse Creek

mation sign on the east side of the north parking area. Good tread
shows that the Strayhorse Creek Trail was once a well-constructed
trail. A single switchback takes you into the densely forested head of
Strayhorse Creek, which is normally dry at this point, and down the
creek to Strayhorse Spring, marked by a ruined log cabin.

Tip: *This spot offers water and the only sizable campsite for the next
several miles.*

As you continue down the creek on the ever-fainter Strayhorse
Creek Trail, take careful note of the tree blazes. These short and long
vertical slashes are the standard Forest Service blazes, and they will
often be your only means of locating the trail. Some of the blazes
along this route are quite fresh, but others have nearly grown over
and can be hard to spot. If you lose the trail, backtrack to the last blaze
and search from there. Although you can't get lost—all you have to
do is follow the creek bed and you'll arrive at the Blue River—the old
trail is usually worth finding. As bad as it is, it will save you energy
compared to thrashing down the creek bed, which is often blocked
with deadfall. Strayhorse Creek flows much of the way, but there are

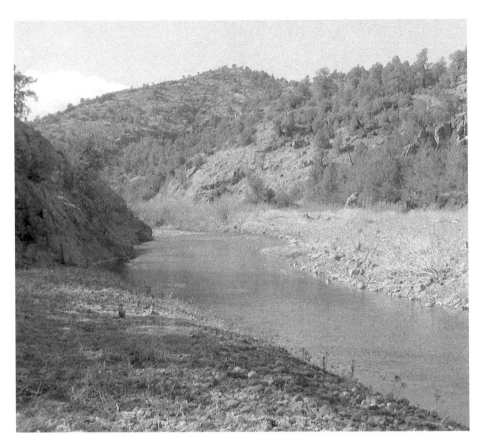

Blue River

almost no camping spots in the upper section of the canyon. You'll do well to average 1.5 miles per hour, but the canyon makes up for the slow going with its beauty and the musical sound of the little creek.

At 4.2 miles from the Rose Peak Trailhead, the creek turns north. As the canyon turns back to the northeast, 1.3 miles further on, an unnamed, major side canyon comes in from the left (west). Below this point, major floods in side drainages buried the trail under debris fans. Some of this flood activity was exacerbated by forest fires, which burned the vegetation cover on the steep slopes above. Another 1.1 miles further downstream, an old sign marks Forest Trail 31, which joins from the left (northwest) (this trail is not shown on the U.S.G.S. topographic map). The Strayhorse Creek Trail improves somewhat after this junction, and the faster going continues past the junction with the Lengthy Canyon Trail (Forest Trail 89), where

Strayhorse Canyon turns east. You'll find numerous campsites on the pine flats along Strayhorse Creek below Lengthy Canyon. Exactly 1.0 mile east of Lengthy Canyon, the ruins of a cabin signal a change in the character of the canyon. Just 0.3 mile downstream of the old cabin, the creek enters a box, or narrows, which is impassable to pack animals. The trail bypasses this section by climbing steeply over a ridge to the north, which is marked with the 5880 spot elevation on the U.S.G.S. map.

Tip: Campsites are rare the next several miles, so you might want to plan on camping before this bypass.

The Strayhorse Canyon Trail becomes much fainter after it plunges down a steep ridge and rejoins the creek.

Tip: From here to the Blue River it is often easier to follow the creek bed.

The trail stays on the alluvial benches along the sides of the creek, crossing at nearly every bend. Deadfall and large amounts of flood debris often choke these benches, but the bed is clear. Precisely 1.0 mile below the box bypass, the canyon opens, the creek disappears underground, and the bed becomes a broad, dry wash. The flow surfaces again just as you reach the Blue River and the Blue River Trail. The old junction is still marked by a Forest Service sign, though little of either trail remains.

Tip: You may have noticed on the maps that the Blue Road, Forest Road 281, ends about two miles to the north. Currently there is no access to the Blue River Trail from the road, due to closure of the old Blue River Trailhead by a private landowner.

Turn right (south) and follow the Blue River downstream. The river, normally a creek-sized flow, swings back and forth across its broad flood plain, and often flows along side rock cliffs at the outside of bends, so you'll find yourself crossing the Blue River at almost every bend. Usually you can hop across on rocks, but you may have to wade. Campsites are plentiful in the Fremont cottonwood and Arizona sycamore groves that line the flood plain. Don't camp near the Blue River, especially during the summer monsoon. The river can quickly flood, as proven by huge piles of debris on the flood plain.

Hike generally south along the Blue River for 5.4 miles to HU Bar Box, a short but dramatic narrows where the Blue River is closely confined by cliffs for a hundred feet or so. You'll have to wade this

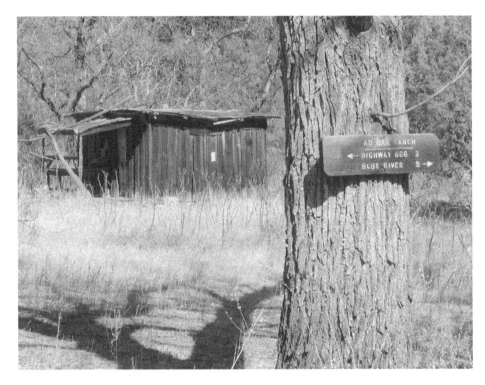

AD Bar Ranch site along AD Bar Trail

section, which is easy when the river is low. While in the narrows, imagine the Blue River in flood, covering the flood plain upstream several feet deep, roaring through the box. Such a flood wrecked a concrete bridge 50 feet above a similar narrows about 11 miles to the north. Just 0.4 mile downstream of HU Bar Box, you'll come to an old cabin on the right bank. The site of the HU Bar Ranch, this old homestead marks the point at which you leave the Blue River.

> **Tip:** *Pick up water from the Blue River, as the next reliable source is 4.6 miles at Rousensock Creek.*

The AD Bar Trail (Forest Trail 14) is not signed. Look for the trail as it crosses a dry wash 100 yards southwest of the ranch buildings. Follow the AD Bar Trail up a steep ridge to the west. Continue on the rocky trail northwest through open pinyon pine and juniper forest and along a grassy ridge top before descending west to cross normally dry Benton Creek. The AD Bar now heads generally southwest, crossing several ridges. At 3.2 miles from the Blue River, the trail descends into dry Thomas Creek and reaches another old homestead cabin, the VT Ranch. You may be able to get water from the old hand-pumped well, which is next to the dry creek bed east of the cabin. The trail now climbs gradually west and passes seasonal Yellow Spring. Follow the AD Bar Trail through a saddle and down a short, steep descent to Rousensock Creek. The creek usually flows at the trail crossing, but there are no campsites. Follow the trail southeast downstream for 0.6 mile and turn southwest up an unnamed tributary to an unnamed saddle. Descend south to Squaw Creek.

Tip: Although the wash is normally dry where the trail meets it, you can find water by walking downstream, past an old corral, toward the unnamed spring marked on the U.S.G.S. map.

Turn right (west), and follow the AD Bar Trail up Squaw Creek. You'll find plenty of campsites in the ponderosa-pine flats along Squaw Creek for the next 1.4 miles upstream, though water only periodically surfaces in the creek.

Follow the AD Bar Trail as it continues west up Squaw Creek. Though the trail is certainly not overused, the going is easy and pleasant compared to the route along Strayhorse Creek. You'll pass the trail's namesake ranch, the abandoned AD Bar, as you continue west. Just 1.0 mile beyond the AD Bar, the trail leaves Squaw Creek and climbs a forested ridge 1.8 miles to the west, to reach U.S. 191 and the trailhead.

Warning: The following itinerary is a minimum. Don't underestimate this hike. Your rate of progress will be slower than usual along Strayhorse Creek and the Blue River.

POSSIBLE ITINERARY

	Camp	Miles	Elevation Gain
Day 1	Spring at head of Strayhorse Creek	5.4	1130
Day 2	Lower Strayhorse Creek	7.5	0
Day 3	Blue River	8.0	0
Day 4	Squaw Creek	8.0	1680
Day 5	Out	4.9	1430

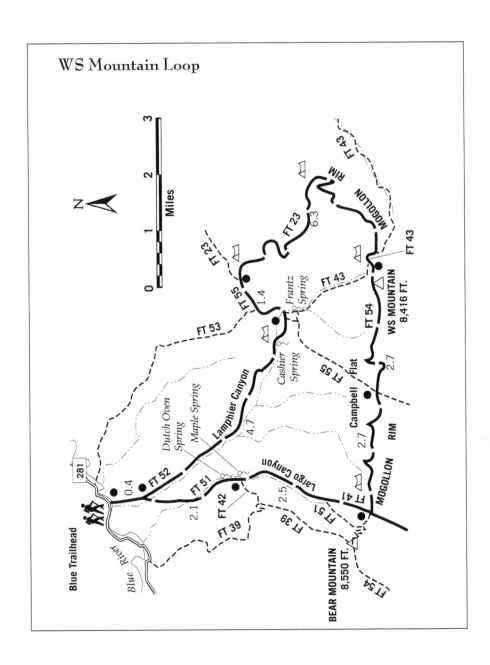

WS Mountain Loop

N

Miles
0 1 2 3

Blue Trailhead

Blue River

281

FT 52 0.4

FT 51

FT 42 2.1

FT 39

FT 51 2.5

Largo Canyon

FT 39

FT 41

Dutch Oven Spring

Maple Spring

Lamphier Canyon 4.7

Cashier Spring

FT 53

FT 55 1.4

Frantz Spring

FT 23

FT 23 6.3

RIM

MOGOLLON

FT 43

FT 43

WS MOUNTAIN 8,416 FT.

FT 54

FT 55

Campbell Flat 2.7

2.7

MOGOLLON RIM

BEAR MOUNTAIN 8,550 FT.

FT 54

13 WS Mountain Loop

RATINGS (1–10)			MILES	ELEVATION GAIN	DAYS	SHUTTLE MILEAGE
Scenery	Solitude	Difficulty	23.8	4220	3	0
7	8	6				

MAPS Bear Mountain, Blue U.S.G.S., Blue Range Primitive and Wilderness Areas U.S.F.S.

SEASON May–November.

BEST June–October.

WATER Seasonal at Lamphier Creek, Cashier Spring, Franz Spring, Tige Spring, Largo Creek, and at Maple and Dutch Oven Springs.

PERMITS None.

RULES None.

CONTACT Alpine Ranger District, Apache-Sitgreaves National Forest, P.O. Box 469 Alpine, Arizona 85920, (928) 339-4384, www.fs.fed.us/r3/asnf.

HIGHLIGHTS This loop takes you through a remote section of the Blue Range Primitive Area. The hike starts by crossing the Blue River, which flows through the heart of the wild area, and then climbs over WS Mountain and traverses a section of the Mogollon Rim through fine stands of ponderosa pine, Douglas-fir, and quaking aspen. From WS Mountain, you'll have outstanding views of the northeastern section of the Blue.

PROBLEMS After a heavy winter, snowdrifts may block the highest section of the loop until late May. The lower sections of this route, near the start and end, are hot during June and July.

HOW TO GET THERE From Alpine, drive 3.2 miles east on U.S. 180 and turn right (south) onto dirt Forest Road 281. Continue 22 miles to the Blue Trailhead on the left (southeast).

DESCRIPTION Follow Forest Trail 52 south across the Blue River. The broad floodplain piled with debris shows the power the Blue River can exert during the spring snowmelt or summer thunderstorms.

> *Warning:* If the Blue River is flooding high, abort the hike and do not attempt to cross the river.

The first 0.3 mile of Forest Trail 52 is on private land. Please stay on the trail and respect private property. On the south side of the Blue River, the trail enters the mouth of Lamphier Canyon, which is vegetated with the pygmy forest of pinyon pine and juniper trees common at this lower elevation. Staying generally on the east side of the creek bed, Forest Trail 52 gradually climbs Lamphier Canyon to the southeast. Just 0.4 mile from the trailhead, watch for Forest Trail 51 on the right (west), which is the return route. Continue south up Lamphier Canyon on Forest Trail 52. For the next 2.2 miles, the trail follows the canyon bottom, where ponderosa pines appear. You may find seasonal water in pools along the creek bed. The trail now climbs away from the bottom of Lamphier Canyon and traverses along a bench several hundred feet above the canyon floor. After 1.4 miles, it drops back to the canyon bottom and passes Cashier Spring.

> *Tip:* You may want to pick up water for camp here, unless there is plenty of water flowing in the creek.

⚜ Wilderness Wildfire

You may notice that much of the country on this loop hike has been burned by recent wildfires. During late summer, you may encounter such fires burning actively but quietly with 1 to 2-foot flames. These naturally occurring fires start from lightning and generally burn at low intensity. Low intensity fires are frequent in undisturbed ponderosa pine forest. Such fires clear out grass, underbrush, and small trees without damaging the fire-resistant large trees, creating an open, parklike forest. This type of fire is beneficial to forest health, and the U.S. Forest Service has developed a policy of letting such fires burn in the Blue unless they threaten structures or people.

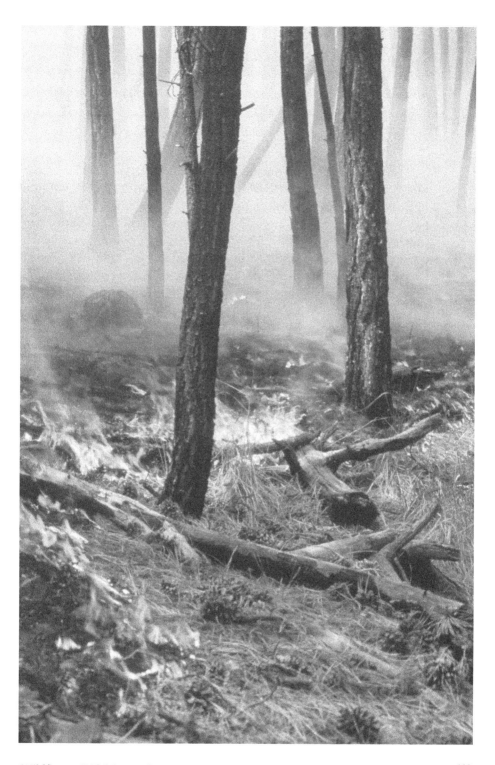

Wildfire on WS Mountain

Beyond the spring, follow Forest Trail 52 onto the south slopes of Lamphier Creek. Head east to the junction with Forest Trail 55, 4.7 miles from the start of the loop. Stay left (east) on Forest Trail 55 and continue another 0.2 mile to Forest Trail 43.

Tip: Franz Spring, 0.2 mile south on Forest Trail 43, is the last reliable water source for the next 14.4 miles.

Turn left (north) on Forest Trail 55 and climb up to Cow Flat. Cow Flat is a broad saddle north of Lamphier Canyon, and the north side of the saddle offers several campsites.

You'll meet Forest Trail 53 just north of Cow Flat. Stay right (northeast) on Forest Trail 55, which contours 0.6 mile on a bench on the north side of Bonanza Bill Point to the junction with Forest Trail 23. Turn right (southeast) on Forest Trail 23 and contour around several tributaries of Tige Canyon. Look for seasonal Tige Spring upstream of the trail in the third tributary. Follow Forest Trail 23 across a fourth tributary of Tige Canyon and south up the fifth tributary to its head at an unnamed saddle on the Mogollon Rim. Here the trail turns sharply west. Climb 700 feet on a series of switchbacks to the northeast rim of WS Mountain. This escarpment on the Mogollon Rim presents spectacular views of the eastern Blue Range. Once on the rim, the trail works its way southwest along gently rolling WS Mountain. Forest Trail 23 ends on top of WS Mountain, 6.0 miles from Forest Trail 55, at the junction with Forest Trail 43.

Continue the hike west on Forest Trail 43 just 0.3 mile to the junction with Forest Trail 54. Here, Forest Trail 43 heads northwest toward Franz Spring and Lamphier Canyon. Stay left and continue west on Forest Trail 54 across the western end of WS Mountain. Forest Trail 54 descends the west end of the mountain to cross Campbell Flat and Forest Trail 55. Camping is plentiful, though you would have to carry water from Cashier, Franz, or Tige Springs, which you passed earlier on the hike.

Continue west on Forest Trail 54 along the Mogollon Rim. The trail climbs over the broad south end of Fire Ridge and descends to another saddle on the Mogollon Rim. A short climb leads over an unnamed hill and into the broad saddle east of Bear Mountain, 5.4 miles from Forest Trail 43. In this unnamed saddle, turn right (north) on Forest Trail 41 and descend into upper Largo Canyon. As the canyon becomes deeper, Forest Trail 41 meets Forest Trail 51 coming in from the left (southwest). Continue north on Forest Trail 51 down Largo

Canyon for 2.5 miles, where Forest Trail 42 comes in on the left, marking the location of Maple Spring. Another water source, Dutch Oven Spring, is 0.3 mile down the canyon. Just 0.9 mile further, Forest Trail 51 leaves Largo Canyon, climbs over the ridge to the east, and descends to end at Forest Trail 52 in Lamphier Canyon, closing the loop. Turn left (north) on Forest Trail 52 and hike north 0.4 mile to the Blue Trailhead.

POSSIBLE ITINERARY

	Camp	Miles	Elevation Gain
Day 1	Cow Flat	6.2	2030
Day 2	Campbell Flat	9.6	1690
Day 3	Out	8.0	500

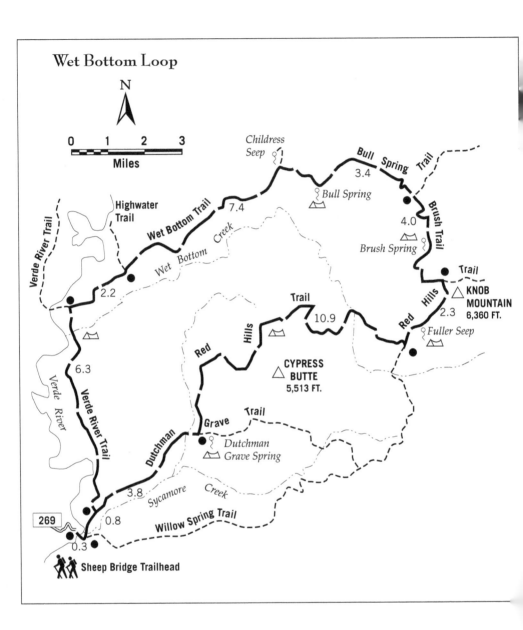

Wet Bottom Loop

N

0 1 2 3
Miles

Highwater
Trail

Wet Bottom Trail 7.4

Childress
Seep

Bull Spring Trail 3.4

Bull Spring

Brush Trail

4.0

Brush Spring

Verde River Trail

Wet Bottom Creek

2.2

6.3

Trail

Trail

10.9

Red Hills

Red Hills

Cypress Butte
5,513 FT.

Knob
Mountain
6,360 FT.

2.3

Fuller Seep

Verde River Trail

Verde River

Dutchman

Grave Trail

Dutchman
Grave Spring

269

3.8

Sycamore Creek

0.8

Willow Spring Trail

0.3

Sheep Bridge Trailhead

14   Wet Bottom Loop

RATINGS (1–10)			MILES	ELEVATION GAIN	DAYS	SHUTTLE MILEAGE
Scenery	Solitude	Difficulty	42.6	7680	5	0
8	7	7				

MAPS Mazatzal Peak, North Peak, Wet Bottom Mesa U.S.G.S., Mazatzal Wilderness U.S.F.S.

SEASON October–April.

BEST October–November, March–April.

WATER Verde River, seasonal at Childers Seep, Bull Spring, Brush Spring, Fuller Seep, Wet Bottom Creek, and Dutchman Grave Spring.

PERMITS None.

RULES The maximum group size is 15 persons and the maximum stay is 14 days.

CONTACT Cave Creek Ranger District, Tonto National Forest, 40202 North Cave Creek Road, Scottsdale, Arizona 85262, (480) 595-3300, www.fs.fed.us/r3/tonto.

HIGHLIGHTS This loop takes you through the rugged Wet Bottom Creek region of the northwestern Mazatzal Mountains. You'll start along the Verde River, a designated Wild and Scenic River within the Mazatzal Wilderness and a rare example of an Arizona desert river. Another segment traverses the East Verde Rim, a north-facing escarpment overlooking the East Verde River and the Mogollon Rim country.

PROBLEMS Some of the trails are little used and can be difficult to follow. You should gain experience on easier trails in the Mazatzal Wilderness before tackling this trip. Carry both the U.S.F.S. wilderness map and the U.S.G.S. topos. All the trails are shown on the U.S.F.S. wilderness map, while the terrain is shown more accurately on the 7.5 minute U.S.G.S. maps. Most of the water sources along this route are seasonal, and may go dry in drought years. Be prepared to carry water for a dry camp, and never depend on a single water source. The desert section of this hike is dangerously hot during the summer months. Mid-winter snow may block the highest section of the loop along the Bull Spring and Brush Trails.

HOW TO GET THERE The Sheep Bridge Trailhead can only be reached via long, rough dirt roads. From the Phoenix area, drive north to Carefree on Scottsdale Road or Cave Creek Road, which meet in Carefree. From Carefree continue northeast on Cave Creek Road. Forest Road 24, a maintained dirt road, continues north after the pavement ends. Precisely 35 miles from Scottsdale Road, turn right on Forest Road 269. Continue 10 miles to the end of the road at the Sheep Bridge Trailhead. The last 5 miles of this road is rough and rocky. Forest Road 24 and Forest Road 269 may become impassable even for high-clearance four-wheel-drive vehicles after a major storm.

You can also reach the junction of Forest Road 24 and Forest Road 269 from Interstate 17 at the Bloody Basin Interchange south of Cordes Junction. Go east on the maintained Bloody Basin Road, which fords the Agua Fria River. This crossing may be impassable when the Agua Fria River is high from snowmelt or a thunderstorm. The Bloody Basin Road turns into Forest Road 269 at the national forest boundary, where it becomes rough. The junction with Forest Road 24 is 25.0 miles from I-17. Continue 10 miles east on Forest Road 269 to the Sheep Bridge Trailhead.

DESCRIPTION From the Sheep Bridge Trailhead, hike east across the Verde River on the Sheep Bridge. After reaching the east bank, turn left (north) onto the Verde River Trail. This trail crosses Sycamore Creek and climbs northeast, away from the Verde River. Exactly 1.1 miles from the trailhead, you'll pass the junction with the Dutchman Grave Trail, the return route. After the junction, the Verde River Trail heads north over a couple of low saddles and descends slightly to cross a desert flat. A short climb leads onto a bluff overlooking the Verde River. The river soon swings away to the west and the trail continues north along a ridge. After the ridge, the Verde River Trail works its way through desert foothills east of the Verde River.

Tip: If you need water, walk west cross-country about a mile. It's easier to carry enough water from the Sheep Bridge Trailhead to reach the crossing of Wet Bottom Creek.

The Verde River Trail crosses Wet Bottom Creek 6.4 miles from the Sheep Bridge Trailhead. This is a good destination for the first day, as most hikers will have spent the morning driving to the trailhead. In spring, Wet Bottom Creek usually flows at the crossing. Otherwise, follow the creek 0.2 mile downstream to the Verde River for water. Campsites are plentiful in the desert flats near the creek.

North of Wet Bottom Creek, the Verde River Trail continues north and climbs onto a ridge, and the Verde River once again swings away to the west. Precisely 1.0 mile from Wet Bottom Creek, turn right (east) onto the Wet Bottom Trail. (The Verde River Trail heads west and crosses the Verde River.) Climb steadily northeast along the ridge north of Wet Bottom Creek for 2.2 miles to the junction with the Highwater Trail. As the name implies, the Highwater Trail serves as an alternate to the Verde River Trail when the Verde River is too high to ford. Continue the main loop on the Wet Bottom Trail northeast along the Sonoran desert ridge. After 2.0 miles, the trail steepens and climbs into high desert grassland. Soon the first dwarf juniper trees start to appear on north-facing slopes, followed by pinyon pines that gradually mix in with the junipers. Sections of the trail may be overgrown with heavy chaparral brush. When the pinyon pine and juniper forest becomes continuous, you have nearly finished the long climb up from the Verde River. After the junction with a spur trail to Childers Seep, the Wet Bottom Trail turns east, passes through a saddle and descends to end at Bull Spring Canyon, 7.4 miles from the Highwater Trail. This delightful spot contains an old rancher's line cabin, a seasonal spring, and plentiful campsites.

The hike continues northeast on the Bull Spring Trail up Bull Spring Canyon. After 1.4 miles, the Bull Spring Trail turns east and climbs out of the brushy basin at the head of Bull Spring Canyon. Follow the trail east along the East Verde Rim, which offers occasional views to the north. After another 2.0 miles, turn right (east) on the appropriately named Brush Trail. (The Bull Spring Trail veers left, diving down Bullfrog Canyon to the East Verde River.) Follow the Brush Trail southeast over Bullfrog Ridge and south into the headwaters of Houston Creek. After hiking 2.0 miles from the start of the

Brush Trail, you'll pass Brush Spring, another seasonal water source with good campsites.

Tip: As with many springs in the Mazatzal Mountains, Brush Spring is shown on the U.S.F.S. wilderness map but not on the U.S.G.S. topographic map.

Follow the Brush Trail southwest up a tributary canyon onto the west end of Knob Mountain, where it ends at the junction with the Red Hills Trail, 2.0 miles from Brush Spring. Turn right (south) on the Red Hills Trail and walk 0.5 mile through the pinyon pine and juniper woodland to the south rim of Knob Mountain and the high point of the loop. Descend steeply southwest on the Red Hills Trail into the Fuller Seep basin, following a series of badly eroded switchbacks. Isolated, scenic Fuller Seep basin is a fine place to camp, and Fuller Seep has seasonal water.

Warning: The sometimes faint Red Hills Trail is not shown on the U.S.G.S. topographic maps. You must have the U.S.F.S. Mazatzal Wilderness map, as well as the topos, to find this trail.

Continue the hike southwest on the Red Hills Trail, and climb 0.6 mile to the junction with the Midnight Trail. Stay right (west) and follow the Red Hills Trail northwest and down to cross Wet Bottom Creek. Normally you'll find water here but there are no campsites. Climb steeply up the Red Hills Trail west of Wet Bottom Creek through a nice stand of red-barked Arizona cypress and onto a ridge.

Tip: The Red Hills Trail from Wet Bottom Creek to the Dutchman Grave Trail is faint in places and makes several sudden changes in direction. The trail is marked with rock cairns. Follow these cairns carefully and do not continue until you have the next cairn in sight.

After the climb, the Red Hills Trail follows a ridge southwest, west, and north, and then suddenly turns west again at a saddle. Descend west down an unnamed tributary of Sycamore Creek 1.6 miles to the confluence of another unnamed tributary. You'll find several campsites and seasonal water at this confluence. Follow the Red Hills Trail south over a broad, unnamed saddle southwest out of the pinyon pine and juniper woodland onto a broad, grassy ridge. Now the trail turns northwest and descends the ridge for 0.9 mile, where the ridge abruptly narrows. Turn southwest and follow the Red Hills Trail down a steep canyon past an old mine. Before reaching the bed of a major unnamed tributary of Sycamore Canyon, turn left (south)

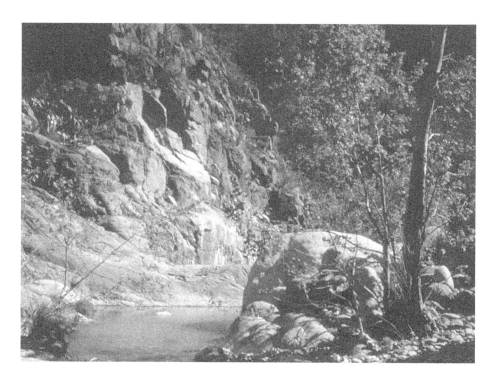

Wet Bottom Creek

and follow the trail along a desert bench and over a saddle. The Red Hills Trail descends to end at the Dutchman Grave Trail, 10.9 miles from the Midnight Trail. You'll find campsites and seasonal water at Dutchman Grave Spring, 0.4 mile east on the Dutchman Grave Trail.

Continue the loop by heading west on the Dutchman Grave Trail southwest over a saddle onto HK Mesa. The trail stays on the top of HK Mesa and heads southwest, meeting the Verde River Trail 3.8 miles from the Red Hills Trail. Turn left here, and return to the Sheep Bridge Trailhead, which is 1.4 miles southwest.

POSSIBLE ITINERARY

	Camp	Miles	Elevation Gain
Day 1	Wet Bottom Creek	6.6	750
Day 2	Bull Basin Spring	10.4	2630
Day 3	Fuller Seep	9.2	2450
Day 4	Dutchman Grave Spring	11.5	1610
Day 5	Out	4.9	240

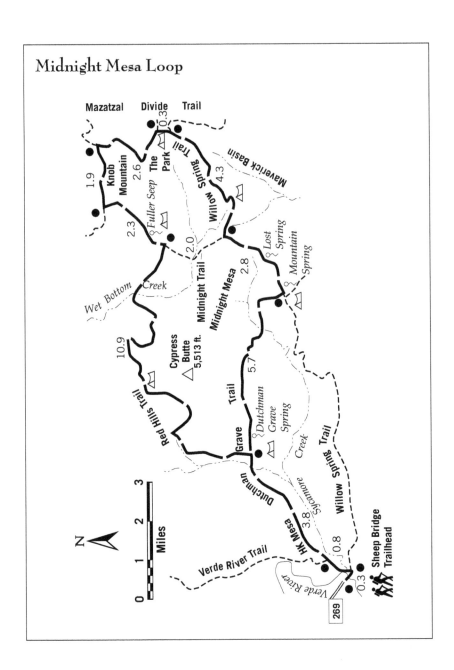

Midnight Mesa Loop

Mazatzal   Divide   Trail

Mazatzal Divide Trail

0.3

1.9

Knob
Mountain

2.6

The
Park

Fuller Seep

Willow Spring Trail

4.3

Maverick Basin

2.3

2.0

Lost
Spring

Mountain
Spring

Midnight Trail

Midnight Mesa

2.8

Wet Bottom Creek

10.9

Cypress
Butte
5,513 ft.

Grave Trail

5.7

Dutchman
Grave
Spring

Sycamore Creek

Willow Spring Trail

Red Hill Trail

Grave

Dutchman

HK Mesa

3.8

0.8

Sheep Bridge
Trailhead

Verde River Trail

Verde River

0.3

269

N

3

2

1

0

Miles

15 Midnight Mesa Loop

RATINGS (1–10)			MILES	ELEVATION GAIN	DAYS	SHUTTLE MILEAGE
Scenery	Solitude	Difficulty	40.6	7650	5	0
8	9	7	(31.2)	(6720)	(4)	

MAPS Cane Springs Mountain, Verde Hot Springs, Wet Bottom Mesa, Chalk Mountain U.S.G.S., Mazatzal Wilderness U.S.F.S.

SEASON October–April.

BEST October–November, March–April.

WATER Verde River, seasonal at Dutchman Grave Spring, Wet Bottom Creek, Fuller Seep, Lost Spring, and Mountain Spring.

PERMITS None.

RULES The maximum group size is 15 persons, and the maximum stay is 14 days.

CONTACT Cave Creek Ranger District, Tonto National Forest, 40202 North Cave Creek Road, Scottsdale, Arizona 85262, (480) 595-3300, www.fs.fed.us/r3/tonto.

HIGHLIGHTS This is a classic loop hike in the western Mazatzal Mountains, starting from cactus-studded desert and looping around Midnight Mesa. The highlight of the trip is the Red Hills Trail, which passes through remote country at the headwaters of Wet Bottom Creek.

PROBLEMS Some of the trails are little used and can be difficult to follow. You should gain experience on easier trails in the Mazatzal Wilderness before tackling this trip. Carry both the U.S.F.S. wilderness map and the U.S.G.S. topographic maps. All the trails are shown on the wilderness map, while the terrain is shown more accurately on the 7.5 minute U.S.G.S. maps. Most of the water sources along this route are seasonal, and may be dry in drought years. Be prepared to carry water for a dry camp, and never depend on a single water source. The desert section of this hike would be dangerously hot during the summer months. Mid-winter snow may block the highest section of the loop along the Mazatzal Divide Trail.

HOW TO GET THERE Bridge Trailhead can only be reached via long, rough dirt roads. From the Phoenix area, drive north to Carefree on Scottsdale Road or Cave Creek Road, which meet in Carefree. From Carefree continue northeast on Cave Creek Road. After the pavement ends, Forest Road 24, a maintained dirt road, continues north. Precisely 35 miles from Scottsdale Road, turn right on Forest Road 269. Continue 10 miles to the end of the road at Sheep Bridge Trailhead. The last 5 miles of this road is rough and rocky. Forest Road 24 and Forest Road 269 may become impassable even for high-clearance four-wheel-drive vehicles after a major storm.

You can also reach the junction of Forest Road 24 and Forest Road 269 from Interstate 17 at the Bloody Basin Interchange south of Cordes Junction. Drive east on the maintained Bloody Basin Road, which fords the Agua Fria River. This crossing may be impassable when the Agua Fria River is high from snowmelt or a thunderstorm. The Bloody Basin Road becomes Forest Road 269 at the national forest boundary, and becomes rougher. The junction with Forest Road 24 is 25.0 miles from I-17. Continue 10 miles east on Forest Road 269 to Sheep Bridge Trailhead.

DESCRIPTION From Sheep Bridge Trailhead, hike east across the Verde River on Sheep Bridge. Just after reaching the east bank, turn left (north) onto the Verde River Trail. This trail crosses Sycamore Creek and climbs northeast, away from the Verde River. Just 1.1 miles from the trailhead, turn right (northeast) on the Dutchman Grave Trail. This trail contours around the south side of a small hill, and then climbs onto the flat expanse of HK Mesa. The Dutchman Grave Trail traverses the length of HK Mesa through desert scrub and cactus and provides frequent views of the rugged mountains ahead.

Tip: Sycamore Creek, a perennial stream, parallels the trail about 0.5 mile to the south. If you need water, you can reach the creek via a short cross-country hike.

At the northeast end of HK Mesa, the trail contours around the south side of a small hill and climbs over an unnamed saddle. After

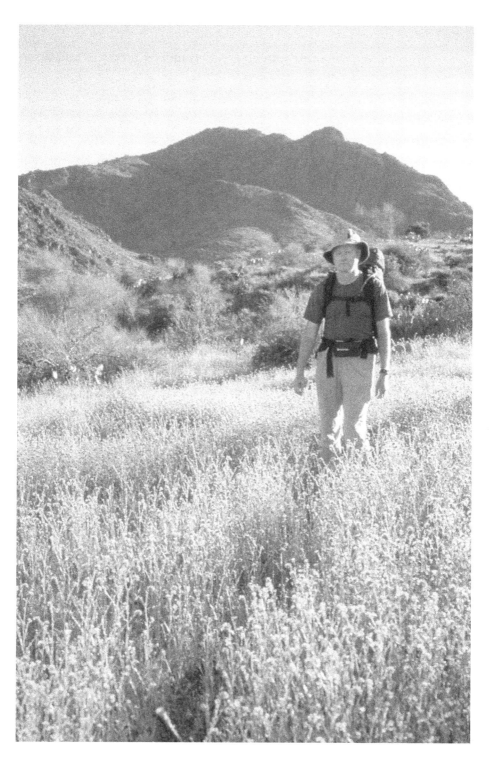

Spring wildflowers on the Dutchman Grave Trail

crossing an unnamed tributary of Sycamore Creek, the trail turns east and meets the Red Hills Trail.

Tip: If it's late in the day, you may want to continue straight ahead 0.5 mile on the Dutchman Grave Trail to Dutchman Grave Spring. This spring is usually reliable and campsites are in the vicinity. The next reliable water is 9.2 miles at the Wet Bottom Creek crossing.

The Red Hills Trail from Dutchman Grave Trail to Wet Bottom Creek is faint in places and makes several sudden changes in direction. The trail is marked with rock cairns. Follow these cairns carefully and do not continue until you have the next cairn in sight.

Turn left (north) on the Red Hills Trail to start the loop section of the trip. After leaving the Dutchman Grave Trail, the Red Hills Trail heads generally north, staying east of a major tributary of Sycamore Creek. After 1.5 miles, the trail veers northeast and climbs a steep side canyon, passing an old mine site. The ascent of this canyon marks the transition from Sonoran desert, with its distinctive stands of giant saguaro cactus, to high desert grassland on the Red Hills. This wild area seems to have received its name from reddish granite outcrops.

Warning: The sometimes faint Red Hills Trail is not shown on the U.S.G.S topographic maps. You must have the U.S.F.S. Mazatzal Wilderness map as well as the topos to find this trail.

At the top of the side canyon, the trail abruptly turns southeast and heads up a ridge toward Cypress Butte. Just 1.0 mile later, the trail turns northeast and climbs along a drainage toward a broad, unnamed saddle into pinyon pine and juniper woodland. From the saddle, the Red Hills Trail descends gradually north along an unnamed tributary of Sycamore Creek and meets another unnamed tributary. You'll find several campsites and seasonal water at this confluence. Follow the Red Hills Trail east up the second unnamed tributary. The trail stays on the north side of the drainage. Exactly 1.6 miles from the confluence, the Reed Hills Trail reaches an unnamed saddle overlooking the deep canyon of Wet Bottom Creek. From the saddle, the trail turns sharply right and climbs a ridge to the southwest, only gradually swinging back to the east as it stays on the highest terrain. After passing hill 5601 (shown on the U.S.G.S. topo), the Red Hills Trail turns northeast and descends a steep ridge through a stand of Arizona cypress trees into Wet Bottom Creek. Deep pools make Wet

Bottom Creek a pleasant lunch stop, but there are no campsites. Follow the Red Hills Trail southeast up a minor, unnamed tributary and south across a ridge into another minor tributary of Wet Bottom Creek. The trail passes through a saddle and turns east to meet the north end of the Midnight Trail, 10.9 miles from the Dutchman Grave Trail and 1.8 miles from Wet Bottom Creek. The Midnight Trail offers an optional shortcut.

To continue the main loop, follow the Red Hills Trail east into the scenic basin at seasonal Fuller Seep. You'll find several campsites near the spring. Climb east up an unnamed tributary of Wet Bottom Creek and up a steep ridge onto the southwest rim of Knob Mountain. Once on top of this mesa, turn north for 0.5 mile to the junction with the Brush Trail, which is 2.3 miles from the Midnight Trail junction.

Tip: *This trail junction and the remainder of the Red Hills Trail are shown incorrectly on the U.S.G.S. topographic map. The U.S.F.S. wilderness map correctly shows the Red Hills Trail passing along the north side of Knob Mountain.*

From the Brush Trail junction, follow the Red Hills Trail east, and contour through the ponderosa-pine stands on the north slopes of Knob Mountain. The Red Hills Trail ends at the junction with the Mazatzal Divide Trail, 1.9 miles from the Brush Trail junction.

Turn right (south) on the Mazatzal Divide Trail and hike around the east end of Knob Mountain. After descending through an unnamed saddle, contour around the head of City Creek and follow the

☀ Pinyon Pine and Juniper Woodland

A miniature, open forest of pinyon pines and juniper trees covers vast tracts of the plateaus and mesas of the Southwest. Several species of juniper trees, sometimes incorrectly called cedars, are predominant in this type of forest. In slightly wetter, more favorable locations, pinyon pines appear with the junipers. Pinyon cones contain an edible nut that is prized by native peoples and newcomers alike. Pinyon jays depend on pinyon nuts for food year round. During the summer and fall, these blue-gray, medium-sized birds fill the pygmy forest with their distinctive calls as they cache pinyon nuts for the winter. After snow falls, pinyon jays demonstrate amazing feats of navigation as they return to their nut caches with an uncanny 90 percent accuracy.

trail southeast into The Park, which is 2.6 miles from the Red Hills Trail. This small ponderosa-pine flat marks the head of Wet Bottom Creek. You'll find plenty of campsites but no water except after wet weather. At the north side of The Park, you'll meet the North Peak Trail. Stay right (south) on the Mazatzal Divide Trail and walk 0.3 mile to the Willows Spring Trail junction, which is just south of The Park. Turn right (south) onto the Willow Spring Trail.

Follow Willow Spring Trail as it contours south and southwest along gentle slopes 1.0 mile to the unnamed saddle at the head of Deadman Creek. (A faint, unmarked trail shown on the topo heading southeast from this saddle is the old route of the Mazatzal Divide Trail.) Continue southwest 2.1 miles on the Willow Spring Trail along a ridge, and down a steep descent to another unnamed tributary of Wet Bottom Creek. You'll find seasonal water and several campsites at this crossing. Head west on the Willow Spring Trail, which contours onto the ridge dividing Wet Bottom and Deadman creeks, to the junction with the south end of the Midnight Trail, 4.3 miles from the Mazatzal Divide Trail.

Turn left (south) and follow the Willow Spring Trail across the east end of Midnight Mesa and down onto a ridge. Cross a broad, unnamed saddle and descend southwest along a drainage past Lost Spring. This seasonal spring is shown on the U.S.F.S. wilderness map but not on the U.S.G.S. topo map. Follow the Willow Spring Trail back onto the ridge crest southwest of the spring and west through an unnamed saddle. Descend west to Mountain Spring and the junction with the Dutchman Grave Trail, 2.8 miles from the Midnight Trail. Mountain Spring appears to be reliable and lies south of the trail at the end of a short spur trail. You'll find a few campsites in the area.

Turn right (northwest) on the Dutchman Grave Trail and contour across a grassy slope.

Tip: Sections of the Dutchman Grave Trail from Mountain Spring to Dutchman Grave Spring are faint—watch for rock cairns marking the route. The trail is shown on the U.S.F.S. wilderness map but not on the U.S.G.S. topographic map.

Just 1.0 mile from the Willow Spring Trail, the Dutchman Grave Trail turns west and descends to cross the head of Sycamore Creek below Granite Basin. Continue west below the south rim of Midnight Mesa and cross several drainages and ridges radiating southwest from Midnight Mesa, before passing through an unnamed saddle. Contour around the north side of hill 4165 (shown on the topo map) and descend onto a gentle slope above Dutchman Grave Spring. As on the outbound section of the trip, Dutchman Grave Spring makes a good campsite. From the spring, walk 0.5 mile west to the junction with the Red Hills Trail, closing the loop 5.7 miles from the Willow Spring Trail. Return to the Sheep Bridge Trailhead the way you came, on the Dutchman Grave and Verde River trails.

POSSIBLE ITINERARY

	Camp	Miles	Elevation Gain
Day 1	Dutchman Grave Spring	4.9	820
Day 2	Fuller Seep	11.5	4110
Day 3	Wet Bottom Creek	9.8	1470
Day 4	Dutchman Grave Spring	9.5	1010
Day 5	Out	4.9	240

MIDNIGHT MESA TRAIL OPTIONAL SHORTCUT The short but scenic Midnight Trail cuts 9.4 miles from the loop, potentially making the trip a day shorter. From the Red Hills Trail/Midnight Trail junction, hike south on the Midnight Trail and descend to Wet Bottom Creek. Seasonal water flows in Wet Bottom Creek, but you'll find few campsites. Climb south 2.0 miles from the Red Hills Trail to meet the Willow Spring Trail. Turn right (south) on the Willow Spring Trail to rejoin the main loop.

Deadman Creek Loop

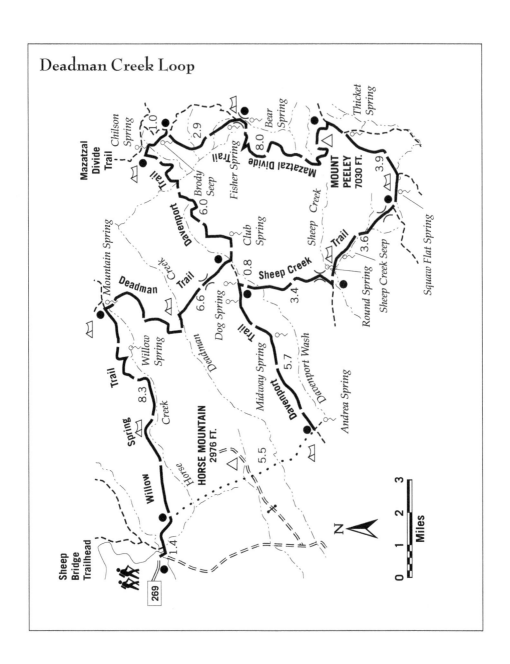

16 Deadman Creek Loop

RATINGS (1–10)			MILES	ELEVATION GAIN	DAYS	SHUTTLE MILEAGE
Scenery	Solitude	Difficulty	57.7	11,510	7	0
7	9	8	(63.6)	(14,680)	(7)	

MAPS Chalk Mountain, Table Mountain, Cypress Butte, North Peak, Wet Bottom Mesa U.S.G.S., Mazatzal Wilderness U.S.F.S.

SEASON October–April.

BEST October–November, March–April.

WATER Verde River, seasonal at Andrea Spring, Midway Spring, Dog Spring, Rock Spring, Round Spring, Sheep Creek Seep, Squaw Flat Spring, Thicket Spring, Bear Spring, Fisher Spring, Brody Seep, Chilson Spring. South Fork Deadman Creek, Club Spring, Mountain Spring, Willow Spring, Horse Creek.

PERMITS None.

RULES The maximum group size is 15 persons, and the maximum stay is 14 days.

CONTACT Cave Creek Ranger District, Tonto National Forest, 40202 North Cave Creek Road, Scottsdale, Arizona 85262, (480) 595-3300, www.fs.fed.us/r3/tonto.

HIGHLIGHTS This long loop hike features a scenic cross-country walk through the Sonoran desert as well as a section of the Mazatzal Divide Trail/Arizona Trail along the pine-forested crest of the Mazatzal Mountains.

PROBLEMS Because a section of the main loop is cross-country, at least one member of the party should have cross-country desert hiking experience. Less experienced groups should do the Willow Spring Trail-Deadman Trail Option, which is entirely on trail. Most of the springs and creeks are seasonal, and may go dry in drought years.

The desert section of this hike is dangerously hot during the summer months. Mid-winter snow may block the highest section of the loop, along the Mazatzal Divide Trail.

HOW TO GET THERE Sheep Bridge Trailhead can only be reached via long, rough dirt roads. From the Phoenix area, drive north to Carefree on Scottsdale Road or Cave Creek Road, which meet in Carefree. From Carefree continue northeast on Cave Creek Road. After the pavement ends, Forest Road 24, a maintained dirt road, continues north. Precisely 35 miles from Scottsdale Road, turn right on Forest Road 269. Continue 10 miles to the end of the road at Sheep Bridge Trailhead. The last 5 miles of this road are rough and rocky. Forest Road 24 and Forest Road 269 may become impassable even for high-clearance four-wheel-drive vehicles after a major storm.

> *Warning:* The main loop has a cross-country section in the desert foothills that requires map and compass skills. A Global Positioning System receiver may also be useful. Do not attempt this loop unless you are comfortable with cross-country hiking in the desert.

You can also reach the junction of Forest Road 24 and Forest Road 269 from Interstate 17 at the Bloody Basin Interchange south of Cordes Junction. Go east on the maintained Bloody Basin Road, which fords the Agua Fria River. This crossing may be impassable when the Agua Fria River is high from snowmelt or a thunderstorm. The Bloody Basin Road becomes Forest Road 269 at the national forest boundary, where it becomes rougher. The junction with Forest Road 24 is 25.0 miles from I-17. Continue 10 miles east on Forest Road 269 to Sheep Bridge Trailhead.

> *Tip:* The Willow Spring Trail-Deadman Trail Option is all on trail, and is strongly recommended for backpackers inexperienced in cross-country travel in the desert. Although it is 5.9 miles longer than the main loop, it is an easier loop.

DESCRIPTION Walk across Sheep Bridge and the Verde River to start the hike. On the east side of the Verde River, follow the Willow Spring Trail across Horse Creek to the junction with the Verde River Trail.

Continue straight (east) on the Willow Spring Trail. Hike east on the trail for about 1.4 miles to where the Willow Spring Trail makes a slight turn northeast. Leave the trail and head cross-country southeast toward the west side of Horse Mountain, 2 miles ahead. The exact point at which you leave the Willow Spring Trail is not critical. If you want to avoid the cross-country section of the loop, stay on the Willow Spring Trail and use the Willow Spring Trail–Deadman Trail option.

Continue the main loop by walking cross-country south-southeast though the open Sonoran desert to a broad drainage that heads west of Horse Mountain. Southwest of Horse Mountain and 2.9 miles from the Willow Spring Trail, you'll cross a two-track road. (This road goes to a line cabin within the wilderness, and is open only to the rancher.) Continue south-southeast, heading toward Andrea Spring. You'll cross Deadman Creek 1.0 mile after crossing the two-track road. Deadman Creek has seasonal water. Andrea Spring is shown correctly on the U.S.F.S. Mazatzal Wilderness Map but is shown without a name on the topo quad. Navigation gets a bit tricky in the low desert foothills as you approach the area of the spring, and close reading of the topographic map is necessary. Your aim is to reach the Davenport Trail, Forest Trail 89, on the ridge where a spur trail goes to Andrea Spring, 1.6 miles from Deadman Creek.

Warning: *The Davenport Trail is faint and receives little use. Don't cross it by mistake.*

Tip: *A GPS receiver, preloaded with the location of the spur trail junction, would be very useful for locating this point.*

This area, 6.9 miles from the Sheep Bridge Trailhead, would be a good goal for a first night's camp.

Head northwest on the Davenport Trail, which climbs along the slopes north of Davenport Wash. The trail heads numerous dry tributaries of Davenport Wash, and climbs over several unnamed saddles as it works its way deeper into the Mazatzal backcountry. Cattle trails may confuse the route; watch for rock cairns marking the official trail. Near the end of the trail, you'll pass Dog Spring, which is shown on the wilderness map but not the topographic map. Turn right on the Sheep Creek Trail, which is 5.7 miles from Andrea Spring. The Sheep Creek Trail heads south and promptly descends to cross Davenport Wash near the end of Mazatzal Wash. Follow the trail, now in high desert grassland, as it climbs over a saddle and drops into Bear Creek. Continue south on the Sheep Creek Trail and ascend an unnamed tributary to an unnamed saddle overlooking Sheep Creek. Descend on the trail to the junction with the Sears Trail, 3.4 miles

In the late 1800s, C. Hart Merriam camped at the foot of San Francisco Mountain in northern Arizona and began a series of explorations of the nearby canyons and mountains. As a result of his research, Merriam developed the concept of life zones. These zones have upper and lower elevation limits and contain an association of plants and animals that are able to flourish in specific climates. Merriam concluded that by going from the bottom of the Grand Canyon to the top of San Francisco Mountain, an elevation gain of 10,000 feet, a traveler would encounter the same range of life zones as a traveler journeying from northern Mexico to northern Canada. While subsequent research points to a variety of other factors, Merriam's basic concept can still help you visualize the progression of life as you hike from the lower Sonoran desert near Sheep Bridge to the transitional ponderosa-pine forest along the crest of the Mazatzal Mountains.

from the Davenport Trail. Follow the Sheep Creek Trail right (east) to the bed of Sheep Creek. After a wet winter, Sheep Creek may be flowing, but otherwise you will have to look for water at Round Spring or Sheep Creek Seep. You'll find a campsite at Round Spring.

Continue the loop on the Sheep Creek Trail, which heads southeast up an unnamed tributary of Sheep Creek. Along this section increasing elevation causes the desert grassland to give way to slopes covered with dense chaparral brush. A steep climb at the head of this drainage brings you to the rim of Squaw Flat, a basin at the head of McFarland Creek. The Sheep Creek Trail continues through pinyon pine and juniper woodland to end at the Copper Camp Trail, 3.6 miles from the Sears Trail junction. Turn left (east) and follow the Copper Camp Trail along McFarland Creek, past Squaw Flat Spring, 0.9 mile to the Thicket Spring Trail.

> **Tip:** You may want to pick up water for a dry camp at Squaw Flat Spring or Thicket Spring. Both of these springs are a bit too close to Sheep Creek for a camp, but if you continue beyond Thicket Spring you'll find no water for 8.8 miles, until Bear and Fisher springs.

Turn left (northeast) on the Thicket Spring Trail, and climb along the brushy southeast slopes of Sheep Mountain to Thicket Spring. Turn left (north) on the Cornucopia Trail and follow this sometimes brushy trail along the east slopes of Mount Peeley 0.8 mile to the

Mazatzal Divide Trail, 3.9 miles from the Sheep Creek Trail-Copper Camp Trail junction. Turn left on the Mazatzal Divide Trail and climb the east slopes of Mount Peeley in several switchbacks. As the trail contours around the north side of Mount Peeley, you'll encounter a ponderosa-pine forest. Follow the Mazatzal Divide Trail south around a tributary of Deer Creek and climb north along the main crest of the Mazatzal Mountains. You'll pass through several saddles on the crest, which offer small campsites but no water. The Mazatzal Divide Trail passes over the highest point of the loop at 7110 feet, turns east and descends to Fisher Saddle, 8.0 miles from the Cornucopia Trail. Fisher Saddle has small campsites. Bear Spring, 0.2 mile south on a spur trail, has seasonal water. As the Mazatzal Divide Trail leaves Fisher Saddle, turn left (north) on the Fisher Trail and descend the headwaters of the South Fork of Deadman Creek past Fisher Spring. Follow the Fisher Trail north across the rugged ridges west of Mazatzal Peak, and ascend to the Brody Trail junction, 2.9 miles from Fisher Saddle. Turn left on the Brody Trail (north), descend past seasonal Brody Seep, and climb north to Chilson Camp and the junction with the Davenport Trail, 1.0 mile from the Brody Trail junction. Chilson Camp, a former rancher's line camp, has plenty of campsites of Mazatzal Peak. Unfortunately Chilson Spring, which is piped down to the camp, is no longer reliable.

Tip: *If you want to spend the night at Chilson Camp, carry water from Fisher Spring or Brody Seep.*

You may have to look carefully for the faint Davenport Trail, which leaves Chilson Camp to the west. Contour west on the Davenport Trail through juniper woodland, around a rock spur, and then descend steeply into the dramatic canyon of the South Fork of Deadman Creek. The scenic creek crossing often has flowing water. A steep but short climb leads out the west side of the canyon, where the ascent moderates as the trail climbs up a tributary and over an unnamed saddle. Descend steadily southwest out of the juniper woodland into high desert grassland. The Davenport Trail turns sharply south and reaches Club Spring in an unnamed tributary of Davenport Wash. This spot is the site of one of the few surviving line cabins in the Mazatzal Mountains. Camping is limited at Club Spring.

Tip: *You may want to pick up water and continue to Deadman Creek for camp.*

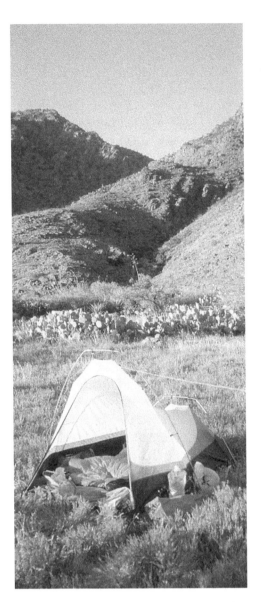

Camp near Willow Spring

Follow the Davenport Trail west and descend to the junction with the Deadman Trail in Davenport Wash, 6.0 miles from Chilson Camp. Turn left (northwest) and follow the Deadman Trail as it climbs steeply to an unnamed saddle northeast of Table Mountain. The trail promptly descends to cross seasonal Deadman Creek. The Deadman Trail may be obscure where it climbs north to an unnamed saddle above Deadman Creek. Turn right and continue climbing to reach the Willow Spring Trail, 6.6 miles from the Davenport Trail junction.

Mountain Spring is apparently reliable, and it is reached by turning right (east) on the Willow Spring Trail. After 0.2 mile, turn right (south) on the 0.1 mile spur trail to the spring. You'll find limited camping in the Mountain Spring area.

Continue the loop from the Deadman Trail junction by turning left (west) on the Willow Spring Trail. Climb west out of the picturesque basin at the head of Horse Creek, cross a ridge, and descend rapidly west down a ridge. The Willow Spring Trail turns abruptly south and descends to an unnamed saddle. You'll find small campsites in the saddle, and a spur trail goes southeast 0.3 mile to Willow Spring. Continue the loop on the Willow Spring Trail, which descends southwest onto a low ridge next to Horse Creek.

Tip: *You may find water in Horse Creek where the trail makes its closest approach to the creek.*

You'll find unlimited camping in the open desert to the west. The final section of the loop follows the Willow Spring Trail as it descends gently westward to Sheep Bridge, 9.7 miles from the Deadman Trail junction.

POSSIBLE ITINERARY

	Camp	Miles	Elevation Gain
Day 1	Andrea Spring	6.9	390
Day 2	Sheep Creek	9.1	2400
Day 3	Mazatzal Divide Trail	10.5	3220
Day 4	Chilson Camp	8.8	1650
Day 5	Deadman Creek	8.2	1330
Day 6	Willow Spring	6.1	2520
Day 7	Out	8.1	0

WILLOW SPRING TRAIL-DEADMAN TRAIL OPTION If you want to avoid the cross-country section of the loop, stay on the Willow Spring Trail to a junction just before Mountain Spring; go right and hike south on the Deadman Trail across Deadman Wash to the Davenport Trail. Turn right on the Davenport Trail and hike 0.8 mile to the Sheep Creek Trail, where you'll turn left, joining the main loop. Look for water at Horse Creek just before the Willow Creek Trail starts its climb to Willow Spring Basin, at Willow Spring, and Mountain Spring. You'll find unlimited camping in the open desert along the Willow Spring Trail until it starts the climb above Horse Creek. Camping for small parties is available on the saddle at the spur trail to Willow Spring and near Mountain Spring.

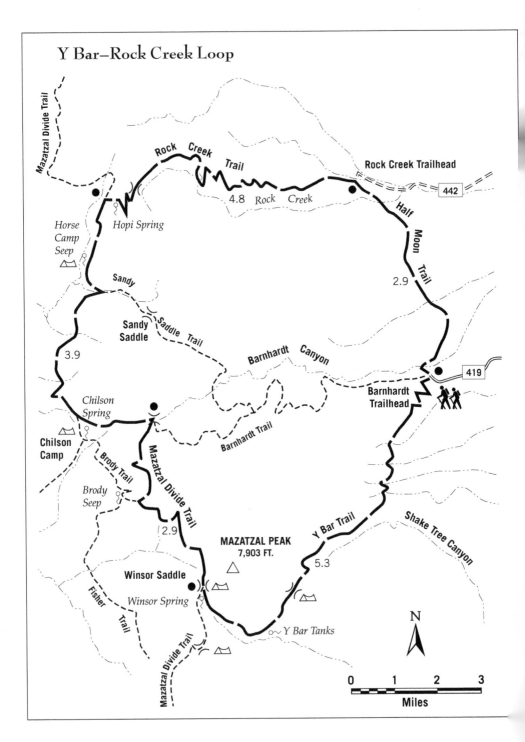

Y Bar–Rock Creek Loop

Mazatzal Divide Trail

Rock Creek Trail

Rock Creek Trailhead

442

4.8 Rock Creek

Half Moon Trail

Horse Camp Seep

Hopi Spring

Sandy

2.9

3.9

Sandy Saddle Trail

Sandy Saddle

Barnhardt Canyon

419

Chilson Spring

Barnhardt Trailhead

Chilson Camp

Brody Trail

Mazatzal Divide Trail

Barnhardt Trail

Brody Seep

2.9

MAZATZAL PEAK 7,903 FT.

Y Bar Trail

Shake Tree Canyon

Winsor Saddle

5.3

Winsor Spring

Fisher Trail

Y Bar Tanks

Mazatzal Divide Trail

N

0   1   2   3
Miles

17 Y Bar–Rock Creek Loop

RATINGS (1–10)			MILES	ELEVATION GAIN	DAYS	SHUTTLE MILEAGE
Scenery	Solitude	Difficulty	19.8	5190	2	0
7	7	6				

MAPS Mazatzal Peak, North Peak U.S.G.S, Mazatzal Wilderness U.S.F.S.

SEASON October–May.

BEST October–November, mid March–mid May.

WATER Seasonal at Y Bar Tanks, Winsor Spring, Brody Seep, Chilson Spring, and Horse Camp Seep, and Hopi Spring.

PERMITS None.

RULES Maximum group size is 15 persons, and the maximum stay is 14 days.

CONTACT Tonto Basin Ranger District, Tonto National Forest, HC02 P.O. Box 4800, Roosevelt, Arizona 85545, (928) 467-3200, and Payson Ranger District, Tonto National Forest, 1009 E. Highway 260, Payson, Arizona 85541, (928) 474-7900, www.fs.fed.us/r3/tonto.

HIGHLIGHTS This is a scenic loop around the highest peak in the range. It passes through a variety of country and offers hundred-mile views in several directions. In the spring, you may be treated to delightful cascades in Rock Creek.

PROBLEMS None of the springs along this route are reliable. Most years you'll find water at one or more springs, but in dry years there may be no water at all along this loop. Make certain you have enough water capacity to carry water for a dry camp. Water is most abundant after a wet winter.

HOW TO GET THERE From Mesa, drive 67 miles north on Arizona 87 and turn left (west) on the Barnhardt Road. Continue 5.0 miles on this maintained dirt road to the Barnhardt Trailhead.

DESCRIPTION This great hike starts on the Y Bar Trail, the southernmost of the three trails that start from this popular trailhead (the Half Moon Trail, the return route, is on the north side of the parking area). Follow the rocky Y Bar Trail as it switchbacks southwest up the broad mesa, wandering through the juniper and pinyon pine forest. After 1.0 mile, the trail reaches the east slopes of Mazatzal Peak and crosses several small canyons before reaching Shake Tree Canyon, 2.0 miles from the Barnhardt Trailhead. Follow the Y Bar Trail into ponderosa-pine forest and up to an unnamed saddle at the head of Shake Tree Canyon, 1.7 miles further. Dry campsites are available at the saddle, though you would have to carry water from the trailhead. Follow the Y Bar Trail southwest down into Y Bar Basin. When the trail levels out, 0.6 mile below the saddle, watch for Y Bar Tanks Spring in a drainage. If this spring is dry, you can often find water by following the drainage downstream a few hundred yards.

> *Tip:* The trail shown heading southwest out of Y Bar Basin on the Mazatzal Peak topographic map no longer exists.

Follow the Y Bar Trail west and northwest up a steady grade through mixed pinyon pine, juniper, and ponderosa pine to Winsor Saddle, 1.0 mile from Y Bar Tanks. You'll find a small campsite here, but Winsor Spring, a few yards southeast of Winsor Saddle, has water only during wet seasons.

> *Tip:* You'll find larger campsites in a broad saddle about a mile south on the Mazatzal Divide Trail.

Turn right (north) on the Mazatzal Divide Trail, which descends slightly and heads across the steep western slopes of Mazatzal Peak. This open slope provides some spectacular views. You can look west across the entire width of the Mazatzal Wilderness to the distant New River and Bradshaw Mountains. Above your right shoulder tower the cliffs of Mazatzal Peak, which at 7903 feet is the highest point in the Mazatzal Mountains. The trail contours around various ridges and canyons emanating from the mountain and passes the junction with the Brody Trail, 1.6 miles from Winsor Saddle.

> *Tip:* Brody Seep is 0.6 mile down this trail, and may have water if you haven't found any so far.

▲▲ Fault Block Mountains

The Mazatzal Mountains are a classic fault block mountain, part of the Basin and Range Geologic Province that covers Arizona south and westof the Mogollon Rim. In this region, north-south trending ranges were created when geologic forces, acting on a continental scale, stretched the earth's crust. Fractures broke the rock, and huge blocks of crust sank to form valleys, while adjoining blocks rose to form mountains. Often the mountain blocks tilted as they rose. The block that formed the Mazatzal Mountains tilted to the west, creating a steep eastern escarpment and a gentler western slope.

Continue the main loop north on the Mazatzal Divide Trail, which contours across brushy south-facing slopes and pine-forested north-facing slopes, to Barnhardt Saddle. This brushy saddle is 1.3 miles from the Brody Trail junction. The Barnhardt Trail goes southeast from the saddle, providing an option for a shorter loop.

Stay left (west) on the Mazatzal Divide Trail to continue the main loop.

Tip: You may find water in the rocky drainage visible to the left (south) below the trail, about 0.5 mile west of Barnhardt Saddle.

Descending gradually, the Mazatzal Divide Trail contours around a hillside and reaches the junction with the Davenport Trail 0.9 mile from Barnhardt Saddle. You can optionally turn left (south) on the Davenport Trail and hike 0.2 miles to Chilson Camp. At this old cowboy line camp, you'll have a picture-window view of the cliff-bound west face of Mazatzal Peak. Water from Chilson Spring is piped down to the camp, but unfortunately this spring is no longer reliable.

Continue north on the main loop, following the Mazatzal Divide Trail around several unnamed tributaries of Deadman Creek. As is typical near the crest of the Mazatzal Mountains, the trail passes through dense chaparral brush on the south-facing slopes and stands of ponderosa pine on the north-facing sections. After hiking 2.0 miles from the Davenport Trail junction, you'll meet the Sandy Saddle Trail junction in a side canyon. The Sandy Saddle Trail is an optional shortcut.

Continue north on the Mazatzal Divide Trail 0.25 mile to the Horse Camp Seep junction. You can optionally follow the Horse

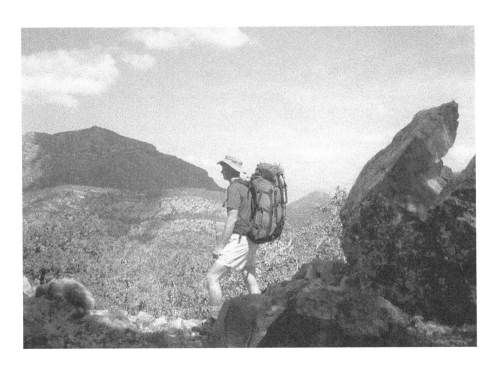

Mazatzal Divide Trail

Camp Seep Trail 0.1 mile north to the seep. There are several campsites under ponderosa pines. The seep is the bed of the North Fork of Deadman Creek west of the campsites. Also, look for water in rock tanks in the bed of the wash just upstream of a 15-foot waterfall. If you have time, follow the wash downstream cross-country 0.25 mile to a view of the deep canyon formed by the headwaters of Deadman Creek.

From the Horse Camp Seep junction, continue the main loop north on the Mazatzal Divide Trail. The trail climbs gradually through mixed pinyon pine, juniper, and ponderosa pine forest to reach the Rock Creek Trail junction and Hopi Spring after 0.8 mile. Water is piped down to a wooden box; if the box is dry, follow the drainage upstream to the actual spring. Turn right (east) on the Rock Creek Trail and climb the brushy slopes along several switchbacks to the an unnamed saddle on the crest of the Mazatzal Mountains. This 7077-foot saddle is the high point of the trip and is 0.8 mile from the Mazatzal Divide Trail. To the west, much of the Mazatzal Wilderness is spread below your feet, and the Mogollon Rim and the Sierra Ancha mountains dominate the view to the east.

Descend the rocky slope to the northeast and follow the Rock Creek Trail south to cross Rock Creek. After the spring snowmelt, Rock Creek contains a delightful cascading creek. The Rock Creek Trail leaves the creek to the north, traverses a narrow ledge under a cliff and descends steeply east along a brushy ridge to reach the Rock Creek Trailhead 4.0 miles from the crest.

At this seldom-used trailhead, turn right (south) on the Half Moon Trail. This relatively new trail is not shown on the U.S.G.S. topographic map. After climbing over a low ridge, the trail works its way across the gently tilted mesas at the foot of the Mazatzal Mountains and ends at the Barnhardt Trail after 2.9 miles.

POSSIBLE ITINERARY

	Camp	Miles	Elevation Gain
Day 1	Chilson Camp	9.3	3030
Day 2	Out	10.5	2160

BARNHARDT TRAIL OPTION From Barnhardt Saddle, you can shorten the loop to 14.3 miles by turning right (southeast) on the Barnhardt Trail. This popular trail descends 1800 feet along the south slopes of impressive Barnhardt Canyon to reach the Barnhardt Trailhead after 6.0 miles.

SANDY SADDLE TRAIL OPTION From the junction with the Mazatzal Divide Trail, you can use the Sandy Saddle Trail to shorten the loop to 18.5 miles. The little-used trail climbs 500 feet over Sandy Saddle on the Mazatzal crest and drops down to cross upper Barnhardt Canyon at unreliable Casterson Seep. It then climbs to meet the Barnhardt Trail, 3.1 miles from the Mazatzal Divide Trail. Turn left (east) on the Barnhardt Trail and descend 4.3 miles to the Barnhardt Trailhead. You'll descend 1800 feet from Sandy Saddle to the Barnhardt Trailhead.

Deer Creek–Y Bar Loop

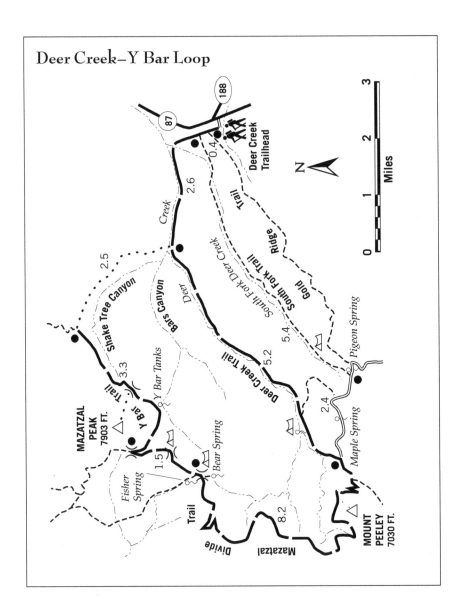

18 Deer Creek – Y Bar Loop

RATINGS (1–10)			MILES	ELEVATION GAIN	DAYS	SHUTTLE MILEAGE
Scenery	Solitude	Difficulty	26.7	4950	3	0
8	8	6	(27.7)	(6930)	(3)	

MAPS Mazatzal Peak U.S.G.S., Mazatzal Wilderness U.S.F.S.

SEASON March–November.

BEST April–May, October

WATER Seasonal at Deer Creek, South Fork Deer Creek, Pigeon Spring, Maple Spring, Bear Spring, Fisher Spring, Winsor Spring, and Y Bar Tanks.

PERMITS None.

RULES The maximum group size is 15 persons, and the maximum stay is 14 days.

CONTACT Tonto Basin Ranger District, Tonto National Forest, HC02 P.O. Box 4800, Roosevelt, Arizona 85545, (928) 467-3200, and Payson Ranger District, Tonto National Forest, 1009 E. Highway 260, Payson, Arizona 85541, (928) 474-7900, www.fs.fed.us/r3/tonto.

HIGHLIGHTS This loop starts from the only Mazatzal trailhead reached from a paved highway. The hike climbs a deep, scenic canyon to the south end of the Mazatzal Divide Trail. The trail winds along the crest of the Mazatzal Mountains and provides 100-mile views of the central mountains. Although this trip can be done as an overnighter, it is much more enjoyable as a three-day trip.

PROBLEMS During the cool season both Deer Creek and the South Fork usually have flowing water. Water is scarce on the Mazatzal Divide Trail. To complete the loop, you'll need to do 2.5 miles of cross-country hiking. Except for a bit of brush at the start, the cross-country section of the route is easy and obvious, and there is an informal trail much of the way.

HOW TO GET THERE From Mesa, drive 63 miles north on Arizona 67. Just south of the junction with Arizona 188, turn left (west) into the Deer Creek Trailhead.

DESCRIPTION Follow the Deer Creek Trail up a single switchback onto a broad ridge. At the top of this ridge, the Gold Ridge Trail branches left (west). Continue north on the Deer Creek Trail down a gentle slope to the junction with the South Fork Trail. The South Fork Trail offers an optional start to the loop.

Continue the main loop on the Deer Creek Trail, which descends into Deer Creek near a windmill belonging to the Deer Creek Ranch. Deer Creek has a seasonal flow during cool weather, and the lower part of the trail is popular with dayhikers. For 2 miles the canyon is fairly open. The rugged Cactus Ridge area is visible high above to the west, which is the area you will traverse at the end of the loop. After you've hiked 3.0 miles from the trailhead, Bars Canyon comes in from the northeast. The cross-country return route descends the grassy ridge to the east of Bars Canyon.

Follow the Deer Creek Trail up Deer Creek to the southwest, climbing gradually up this long canyon. You'll be in pinyon pine and juniper woodland for the first several miles, with chaparral brush dominating on the south-facing, right-hand slope. As you gain elevation you'll notice ponderosa pines appearing on the north-facing slopes. Exactly 1.0 mile after a major tributary comes in from the right, you'll enter a brushy meadow marked Winsor Camp on the U.S.G.S. topographic map.

> *Tip:* The next campsites are 4.1 miles farther, and the next water is 9.3 miles at Bear Spring.

Just above Winsor Camp, the Davey Gowan Trail turns left (east). Stay right (southwest) on the Deer Creek Trail, which continues up Deer Creek another 0.7 mile. A short, steep ascent leads to the end of the Deer Creek Trail at the Mount Peeley Trailhead, 1.1 miles from Winsor Camp.

Follow the Mazatzal Divide Trail west. After 0.5 mile, the Mazatzal Divide Trail meets the junction with the Cornucopia Trail. Follow the Mazatzal Divide Trail west up several switchbacks on the brushy east slopes of Mount Peeley. As you climb, you'll gain a superb view of the headwaters of Deer Creek. After the last switchback, follow the trail across the pine-forested north slopes of Mount Peeley. Optionally, you can leave the trail here and hike to the top of Mount Peeley.

Continue the loop by following the Mazatzal Divide Trail west as it contours around the headwaters of Deer Creek. The trail turns north where it passes through an unnamed saddle and joins the crest of the range. Several saddles along this section offer the first possible campsites since leaving Deer Creek, but they are limited in size and you will have to carry water from Deer Creek. The Mazatzal Divide Trail climbs steadily north and generally

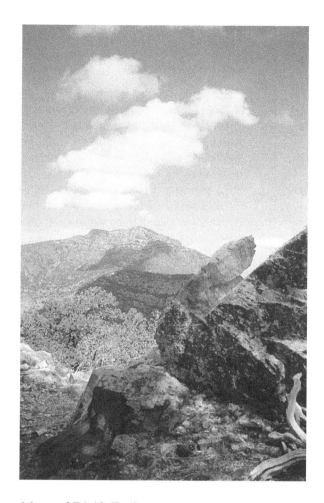

Mazatzal Divide Trail

stays on the east side of the crest. One section of the trail traverses west-facing slopes, offering you a view of the southwestern Mazatzal Wilderness from the crest to the Verde River. The Mazatzal Divide Trail passes through another unnamed saddle and turns west, crossing the 7110-foot summit of the loop. Follow a single switchback down into toward Fisher Saddle, 8.2 miles from the Mount Peeley Trailhead. You'll find a few small campsites in Fisher Saddle, and larger campsites 1.0 mile north on the Mazatzal Divide Trail where it passes through another saddle. Spur trails lead to both Bear Spring,

☼ Chaparral Brushlands

Chaparral is not a plant. It's a close, perhaps too close, association of three shrubs: mountain mahogany, shrub live oak, and manzanita. These tough plants grow in densely intertwined stands covering entire hillsides at elevations of 4000 to 6000 feet in the Mazatzal Mountains and other central Arizona ranges. Reaching heights of 4 to 6 feet, these brushlands are not fun places to hike cross-country, except maybe to build character. Nevertheless, the heavy brush provides excellent cover for wildlife and reduces erosion from heavy summer thundershowers. Cottontail rabbits find the dense cover ideal, and you'll almost certainly hear the beautiful descending trill of the canyon wren.

0.2 mile south of Fisher Saddle, and Fisher Spring, 0.2 mile north and 500 feet below the saddle.

Tip: *Plan to camp near Fisher Saddle because there is little camping beyond this area.*

From Fisher Saddle, follow the Mazatzal Divide Trail north 1.5 miles through an unnamed saddle to Winsor Saddle. You'll find a small campsite here, but Winsor Spring is usually dry. Turn right (southeast) on the Y Bar Trail, and descend into Y Bar Basin. At the low point of this trail, you'll cross a drainage at seasonal Y Bar Tank Spring.

Tip: *If the spring is dry, walk downstream about 100 yards to a series of large rock tanks.*

It is 6.3 miles to the next water source at Deer Creek.

From Y Bar Tanks, follow the Y Bar Trail northeast up to the unnamed saddle between Cactus Ridge and Mazatzal Peak. You'll find campsites in the saddle but no water.

Optionally, you can leave the trail and do a side hike to Mazatzal Peak.

Continue on the loop along the Y Bar Trail down into Shake Tree Canyon, a tributary of Deer Creek. At first, the trail descends through pine forest, but after 1.1 miles the Y Bar Trail comes out onto an east-facing, brushy slope. Below you, Shake Tree Canyon abruptly veers east and cuts dramatically through a fin of purplish Mazatzal quartzite. After passing above this feature, the trail crosses the first of several ridges that descend to the east. Leave the Y Bar Trail on the first ridge, and descend east. The first 0.2 mile is somewhat brushy, but the walking is easy as you descend the grassy slope. Stay on the ridge directly north of Shake Tree Canyon and follow it 2.5 miles to its end at Deer Creek. While the ridge is cross-country, you'll probably find traces of an old trail. Cross Deer Creek and join the Deer Creek Trail on the south side. Turn left (east) and follow the Deer Creek Trail 3.0 miles to the Deer Creek Trailhead.

POSSIBLE ITINERARY

	Camp	Miles	Elevation Gain
Day 1	Upper Deer Creek	7.2	1500
Day 2	Fisher Saddle	9.2	2650
Day 3	Out	10.3	800

SOUTH FORK OPTION From the junction of the South Fork and Deer Creek Trails, turn left (west) on the South Fork Trail. Except for a short excursion onto the south slopes, the South Fork Trail stays near the bed of the seasonal creek, 5.4 miles to the end of the trail at the Mount Peeley Road. Turn right (west) and follow the Mount Peeley Road 2.4 miles to Mount Peeley Trailhead, where you rejoin the main loop. You may find seasonal water in the lower South Fork, and at Pigeon Spring at the upper end of the trail.

Tip: Pick up water along the lower South Fork, because the upper section of the canyon may be dry, and there are no campsites near Pigeon Spring.

MOUNT PEELEY OPTIONAL SIDE HIKE Leave the Mazatzal Divide Trail on the north slopes of Mount Peeley and climb south, cross-country, about 0.3 mile and 600 feet to the rounded summit of Mount Peeley. This 7030-foot summit has a panoramic view of much of the central Mazatzal Mountains and the southern section of the wilderness.

MAZATZAL PEAK OPTIONAL SIDE HIKE From the unnamed saddle between Cactus Ridge and Mazatzal Peak, leave the Y Bar Trail and climb Mazatzal Peak via its southeast ridge. This somewhat brushy cross-country hike ascends 1600 feet in 0.7 mile, and takes you to 7903-foot Mazatzal Peak, the highest point in the Mazatzal Mountains.

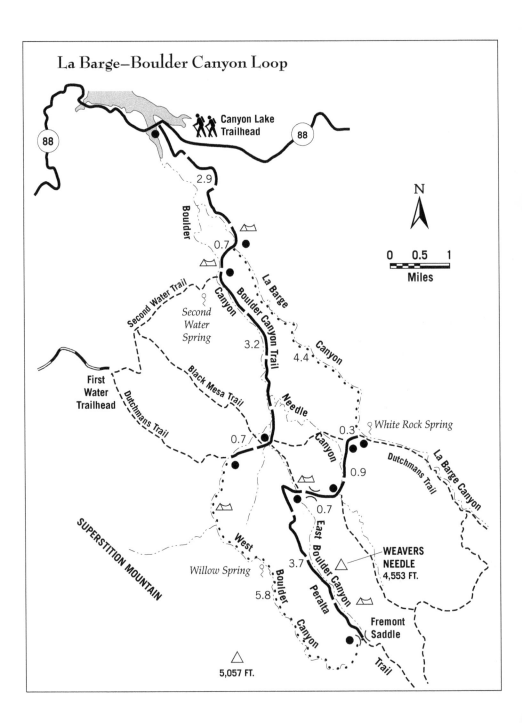

La Barge–Boulder Canyon Loop

88

Canyon Lake Trailhead

88

2.9

Boulder

0.7

Second Water Trail

Boulder Canyon Trail

La Barge

Canyon

Second Water Spring

3.2

Canyon

4.4

First Water Trailhead

Black Mesa Trail

Dutchmans Trail

Needle

White Rock Spring

0.3

0.7

Canyon

0.9

Dutchmans Trail

La Barge Canyon

0.7

SUPERSTITION MOUNTAIN

West

Willow Spring

3.7

Boulder

5.8

Canyon

Peralta

East Boulder Canyon

WEAVERS NEEDLE 4,553 FT.

Fremont Saddle

Trail

5,057 FT.

N

0   0.5   1
Miles

19 La Barge–Boulder Canyon Loop

RATINGS (1–10)			MILES	ELEVATION GAIN	DAYS	SHUTTLE MILEAGE
Scenery	Solitude	Difficulty	26.2	3840	3	0
8	4	6				

MAPS Weavers Needle, Goldfield, Mormon Flat Dam U.S.G.S., Superstition Wilderness U.S.F.S.

SEASON October–April.

BEST Mid October–March.

WATER La Barge Canyon, White Rock Spring, West Boulder Canyon, Willow Spring, and seasonally in East Boulder Canyon and Boulder Canyon.

PERMITS None.

RULES Maximum group size 15 persons and maximum stay limit of 14 days.

CONTACT Mesa Ranger District, Tonto National Forest, 26 N. MacDonald, P.O. Box 5800, Mesa, Arizona 85211-5800, (480) 610-3300, www.fs.fed.us/r3/tonto.

HIGHLIGHTS The La Barge-Boulder Canyon Loop traverses three forks of the spectacular La Barge and Boulder Canyon system in the western Superstition Mountains. The hike mixes on-trail and cross-country hiking and takes you past the most famous Superstition landmark, the twin spires of Weavers Needle.

PROBLEMS Do not attempt this hike during or immediately after a period of heavy rain because the canyons may be flooded and impassable. Water is scarce on this loop during dry periods.

Warning: This hike is extremely hot and dangerously dry during the summer.

HOW TO GET THERE From Apache Junction at the east side of the greater Phoenix area, drive northeast 14.5 miles on Arizona 88 to Canyon Lake Marina, and turn left (north) into the designated trailhead parking.

DESCRIPTION Cross the highway and follow the Boulder Canyon Trail south up the desert slopes. As you climb, a panoramic view of Canyon Lake and the rugged terrain around it opens behind you; don't forget to take a break and look back! You're hiking through classic Sonoran desert, and such distinctive plants as the giant saguaro cactus, and green-barked palo verde trees dominate the landscape. As you continue the ascent, La Barge Canyon opens below you to the west.

After the Boulder Canyon Trail turns east to contour around a side canyon, it climbs over a low ridge and descends steeply to La Barge Creek, 2.4 miles from the trailhead. By now you've hiked far enough to leave the casual dayhikers behind, and the sights and sounds of the busy Canyon Lake recreation area have faded. La Barge Creek flows during the winter and spring, and even in dry periods you will probably find pools. Follow the Boulder Canyon Trail 0.5 mile up the east side of the creek.

Leave the trail where it crosses La Barge Creek and hike cross-country upstream. Hiking up the gravel and boulder strewn wash is easy at first, but as the towering volcanic canyon walls close in, the stream course becomes more restricted. You'll encounter a section of jumbled boulders that takes a while to work through. Named "La Barge Canyon" on the old Goldfield U.S.G.S. map, this narrow canyon is also known as "Lower La Barge Box."

Normally, the term "box canyon" refers to a canyon that "boxes up," or becomes impassable, usually because of a pour off or dry waterfall. In the Superstition Mountains, the term "box" is used to refer to a narrow section of a canyon. Lower La Barge Box, on this hike, is probably impassable to horses but is an enjoyable hike for foot travelers.

After 2.0 miles you'll emerge into March Valley and meet the Cavalry Trail coming in from the west. Follow the faint and little used Cavalry Trail south along Marsh Valley. Low hills border the valley on the west and the cliffs of Peters Mesa dominate the eastern skyline. At the south end of Marsh Valley, you'll meet the well-used Dutchmans Trail.

The Peralta Trail was named for the Peralta family, who reputedly had a gold mine somewhere in the Superstition area in the 18th century, when Arizona was a Spanish colony.

Fremont Saddle is one of many western landmarks named after John C. Fremont. Fremont headed one of several U.S. government surveys sent to the American West after the United States acquired much of the Southwest from Mexico.

Tip: White Rock Spring is located northeast of the junction, but camping is limited.

Turn right (west) on the Dutchmans Trail and hike 0.3 mile to the Bull Pass Trail.

Tip: The old U.S.G.S. map shows the Bull Pass trail incorrectly as the continuation of the Dutchmans Trail.

Stay left (south) on the Dutchmans Trail and follow it south up Needle Canyon for another 0.9 mile to the junction with the Needle Canyon Trail. Turn right (west) and follow the Dutchmans Trail over Upper Black Top Mesa Pass and down into East Boulder Canyon and the Peralta Trail. This beautiful spot, 1.9 miles from the Cavalry Trail, is a good place to camp, and you'll find seasonal water in the creek.

Continue the loop by turning left (west) onto the Peralta Trail and climbing over an unnamed saddle south of Palomino Mountain.

Tip: The old U.S.G.S. map shows trails that no longer exist in this area, and names others incorrectly. The U.S.F.S. wilderness map correctly depicts the trails.

From the unnamed saddle, follow the Peralta Trail south-south-east to another unnamed saddle west of a rocky knob. Contour south into the head of East Boulder Canyon, passing west of towering Weavers Needle, and follow the Peralta Trail as it climbs to Fremont Saddle.

Leave the Peralta Trail and hike cross-country 0.3 mile south up the slope to the top of the ridge. You'll have to work your way around numerous rock pinnacles and small cliffs, but it's easier than it looks.

☀ Sonoran Desert

The western Superstition Mountains are covered by a plant and animal community called Sonoran desert scrub. This desert community extends south into the Mexican state of Sonora. Because the Sonoran desert gets a significant amount of winter and summer rain, it's relatively lush for a desert. The landmark plant is the giant saguaro cactus, which grows with a mixture of desert trees such as palo verde, mesquite, and ironwood. Javelina, a pig-like animal, roams the desert in large bands of up to 20 animals. They can survive for days without water, and eat the succulent pads of the prickly pear cactus, spines and all, for both food and water. Reptiles are a common sight, especially lizards and rattlesnakes. More rare is the Gila monster, a foot-long venomous lizard whose red and black markings clearly say "Leave me alone!"

Tip: The U.S.G.S. topographic map, though sadly out of date as far as the trails are concerned, will be useful in finding your way on the cross-country portions of this loop.

The exact point at which you reach the ridge is not important. From the top of the ridge, turn southwest and descend into the head of West Boulder Canyon. In wet years, you'll find water in pools near the head of the canyon, but in drought years you may have to carry water for camp. As the canyon deepens, you may find sections of the old West Boulder Trail shown on the U.S.G.S. topographic map. You'll find seasonal water at Willow Spring, about midway through the canyon. After Old West Boulder Canyon comes in from the west, the main canyon gradually opens up, and you'll find plenty of camp-sites in the next 1.5 miles.

Tip: To avoid the crowds along the Dutchmans Trail, plan to camp before reaching the trail.

As West Boulder Canyon opens into a broad wash and reaches the base of Black Mesa, it turns northeast. After 5.8 miles of cross-country hiking from Fremont Saddle, you'll meet the Dutchmans Trail as it crosses the broad wash.

The pinnacles that you hike through on the cross-country hike from Fremont Saddle to West Boulder Canyon are the "stone ghosts" of the Superstition Mountains. Apache Indian legend says that the stone ghosts are people who were petrified after a great flood. Geologically, the stone ghosts are rhyolite, a rock formed from volcanic ash.

Turn right (east) on the Dutchmans Trail, and follow it east as it parallels the wash. The trail enters Boulder Basin, a broad, relatively open valley at the confluence of West Boulder, Little Boulder, and East Boulder canyons. Stay right (east) at the junction with the Black Mesa Trail. Just 0.7 mile from where you stepped onto the Dutchmans Trail, turn left (north) on the Boulder Canyon Trail. Follow the Boulder Canyon Trail north down East Boulder Canyon. After 0.4 mile, West Boulder Canyon joins from the left to form Boulder Canyon. Watch for Needle Canyon, a narrow canyon entering from the right. Unless a recent major flood has destroyed it, you'll find a good trail 3.2 miles down Boulder Canyon to the Second Water Trail junction.

Tip: *During the cool season, you should find water at the Second Water Trail junction. If not, hike left (west) up the Second Water Trail to Second Water Spring.*

Continue the main loop by following the Boulder Canyon Trail to the north for 0.3 mile and leave Boulder Canyon to the east. The trail climbs over the unnamed, low saddle north of Battleship Mountain. Follow the Boulder Canyon Trail down into La Barge Canyon to the point where you left it to start the cross-country hike up La Barge Canyon; stay on the trail to retrace your steps 2.9 miles to the Canyon Lake Trailhead.

POSSIBLE ITINERARY

	Camp	Miles	Elevation Gain
Day 1	East Boulder Canyon	9.2	1580
Day 2	West Boulder Canyon	9.1	1740
Day 3	Out	7.9	520

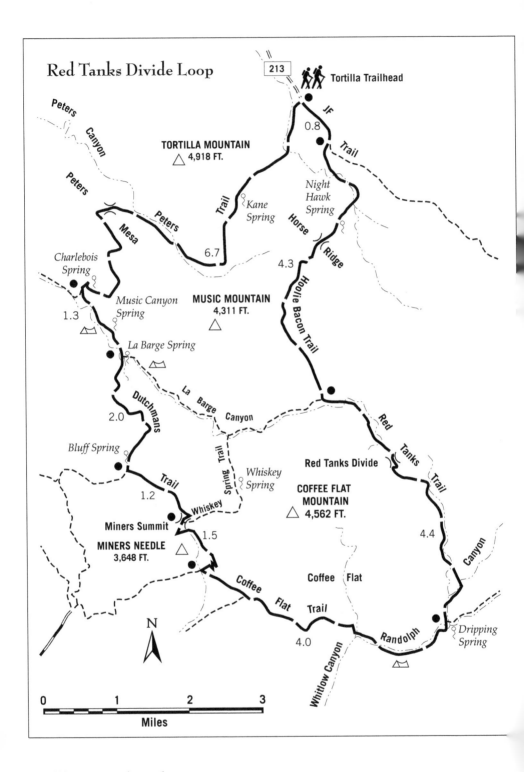

Red Tanks Divide Loop

213

Tortilla Trailhead

JF
0.8

TORTILLA MOUNTAIN
△ 4,918 FT.

Peters

Canyon

Peters

Peters

Mesa

Trail

Kane
Spring

Night
Hawk
Spring

Horse

Ridge

Hoolie Bacon Trail

6.7

4.3

Charlebois
Spring

Music Canyon
Spring

MUSIC MOUNTAIN
4,311 FT.
△

1.3

La Barge Spring

La Barge

Canyon

Red

Tanks

Trail

2.0

Dutchmans

Spring Trail

4.4

Bluff Spring

Trail

Whiskey
Spring

Red Tanks Divide

COFFEE FLAT
MOUNTAIN
△ 4,562 FT.

1.2

Whiskey

1.5

Miners Summit

MINERS NEEDLE
3,648 FT. △

Coffee

Flat

Trail

Coffee Flat

Canyon

4.4

N

Coffee Flat Trail

Randolph

Dripping
Spring

4.0

Whitlow Canyon

0   1   2   3
Miles

20 Red Tanks Divide Loop

RATINGS (1–10)			MILES	ELEVATION GAIN	DAYS	SHUTTLE MILEAGE
Scenery	Solitude	Difficulty	26.2	4360	3	0
8	6	5				

MAPS Mormon Flat Dam, Weavers Needle, Goldfield U.S.G.S., Superstition Wilderness U.S.F.S.

SEASON September–May.

BEST Mid October–March

WATER Seasonal at Night Hawk Spring, Upper La Barge Box, Dripping Spring, Bluff Spring, La Barge Spring, Music Spring, Charlebois Spring, and Kane Spring.

PERMITS None.

RULES Maximum group size 15 persons and maximum stay limit of 14 days.

CONTACT Mesa Ranger District, Tonto National Forest, 26 N. MacDonald, P.O. Box 5800, Mesa, Arizona 85211-5800, (480) 610-3300, www.fs.fed.us/r3/tonto.

HIGHLIGHTS The Red Tanks Divide Loop takes you through a remote section of the Sonoran desert in the headwaters of La Barge and Red Tanks canyons. Using a section of the popular Dutchmans Trail at the midsection, the hike finishes by climbing over a high ridge with good views of the central Superstition Mountains.

PROBLEMS Water sources are far apart at the beginning and end of the loop. All the springs are seasonal, and they may be dry in the fall or after a dry winter. On the other hand, if the winter rains are plentiful, every creek will be running and the spring flowers will be in full bloom.

HOW TO GET THERE Starting from Apache Junction at the east side of the greater Phoenix area, drive 22.3 miles east on Arizona 88. Continue past the end of the pavement and turn right (south) on Tortilla Road, Forest Road 213. Drive 2.9 miles to the Tortilla Trailhead. You'll need a high-clearance, four-wheel-drive vehicle on Forest Road 213. Hikers with low-clearance vehicles will have to hike the road, which adds 5.8 miles to the hike.

Warning: Some of the trails on this loop are little traveled and may be hard to follow. You must have the U.S.F.S. Superstition Wilderness map as well as the U.S.G.S. topographic maps to follow this route. The trails are shown accurately on the wilderness map, but at reduced scale. The U.S.G.S. topos show the terrain in great detail, but many of the trails depicted no longer exist.

DESCRIPTION From the Tortilla Trailhead, hike southeast on the JF Trail as it ascends a desert ridge. After 0.8 mile, turn right (south) onto the Hoolie Bacon Trail and descend into Tortilla Creek. Follow the trail up Tortilla Creek to the southeast. Tortilla Creek is usually a dry wash, but you may find water here after a wet winter. The Hoolie Bacon Trail leaves Tortilla Creek 1.1 miles from the JF Trail, shortly after turning south again. The U.S.G.S. topographic map shows an old trail going to Dogie Spring and Cedar Basin, but this route is no longer maintained and is difficult to find. Stay on the Hoolie Bacon Trail as it climbs south up a drainage past seasonal Night Hawk Spring. Cross over Horse Camp Ridge and descend gradually into Horse Camp Basin. Again, the U.S.G.S. topo shows a trail that no longer exists—the connection to the Peters Trail to the northwest.

From Horse Camp Basin, follow the Hoolie Bacon Trail southeast 0.5 mile down the wash above Trap Canyon. When the wash turns southwest toward Trap Canyon, the Hoolie Bacon Trail leaves the wash and climbs southeast to an unnamed low pass next to Herman Mountain. Follow the trail south to the junction with the Red Tanks Trail at La Barge Canyon, 3.2 miles from Tortilla Creek.

Turn left (east) on the Red Tanks Trail and follow it up La Barge Creek 0.5 mile, where the trail turns right (south) up an unnamed tributary of La Barge Creek.

Tip: You may find pools of water along this drainage where bedrock is exposed.

⚘ Teddy Bear Cholla

This cuddly-looking cactus appears to be covered with fuzzy yellow balls of fur. Those unfortunate enough to touch one of these fuzzy balls find out quickly that they consist of sharp spines with invisible barbs. The balls, or burrs, cling tenaciously to skin, clothing, or boots, and break off easily from the plant. Burrs that land in favorable conditions after their unwilling host gets rid of them germinate new cholla plants.

Use a comb or a pair of sticks to remove the burrs, and then pick out the spines with a good pair of tweezers.

The Red Tanks Trail, faint in places, continues south. It climbs through rolling desert terrain and tops out at Red Tanks Divide, an obscure pass on the complex ridge dividing the Randolph and La Barge Canyon drainages. The view from Red Tanks Divide is dominated by the cliffs of Coffee Flat Mountain. Follow the The Red Tanks Trail down an unnamed tributary into Red Tanks Canyon. The trail continues south along Red Tanks Canyon until near the canyon's end, where the trail climbs out of the bed on the left (east). The Red Tanks Trail climbs over a low ridge and descends into Randolph Canyon just east of the mouth of Red Tanks Canyon. You may find water in the narrows at the lower end of Red Tanks Canyon. After a wet winter, both canyons are often flowing. Follow the Red Tanks Trail southwest and south down Randolph Canyon to the Coffee Flat Trail junction, 4.4 miles from the end of the Hoolie Bacon Trail. This is also the mouth of Fraser Canyon and the location of Dripping Spring, a fairly reliable water source.

Tip: In dry years, pick up water here for camp, as the next possible spring is Bluff Spring, about 7 miles farther.

Turn right (west) on the Coffee Flat Trail and follow it down Randolph Canyon. As you proceed, the canyon floor opens up and you'll find numerous campsites. At Reeds Water, a spot marked by an old windmill, the Coffee Flat Trail turns right and heads north up Coffee Flat Canyon. After 0.1 mile, the trail turns left (west) and climbs over an unnamed low pass to Whitlow Canyon. Follow the Coffee Flat Trail as it climbs gradually northwest over another unnamed low pass. Stay right on the Coffee Flat Trail at the junction with the

Barkley Trail. Continue northwest to the Dutchmans Trail junction, 4.0 miles from the Red Tanks Trail.

Turn right (northwest) on the Dutchmans Trail and follow it 1.6 miles up the east slopes of Miners Canyon to Miners Summit and the Whiskey Spring Trail junction. Stay left (northwest) on the Dutchmans Trail and descend into an unnamed tributary of Bluff Spring Canyon. You'll reach the Bluff Spring Trail junction 1.2 miles from Miners Summit. Remain on the Dutchmans Trail and continue 0.9 mile down Bluff Spring Canyon to the north, where the trail turns west and climbs out of the canyon. The Dutchmans Trail gradually descends to the mouth of Bluff Spring Canyon at the confluence with La Barge Canyon and the junction with the Red Tanks Trail, 2.0 miles from the Bluff Spring Trail. You'll find several campsites and La Barge Spring near this junction. In wet years La Barge Canyon may have plenty of water flowing down it, possible enough to make crossing difficult.

Tip: Look for a campsite before reaching Charlebois Spring, which is heavily used.

Continue northwest on the Dutchmans Trail down La Barge Canyon. A 0.2-mile spur trail goes east to Music Canyon Spring. Staying on the Dutchmans Trail, you'll reach Charlebois Spring and the junction with the Peters Trail 1.3 miles from La Barge Spring. Avoid camping at this overused spot, if possible.

Warning: In dry years, it is 5.1 miles to the next water source at Kane Spring.

Turn right (south) on the Peters Trail and climb steeply onto an unnamed ridge. Follow the trail east and north onto an unnamed ridge, where the trail may become faint. The Peters Mesa Trail is shown accurately on both the U.S.F.S. wilderness map and the U.S.G.S. topographic map. After climbing to the head of an unnamed tributary of Music Canyon, the Peters Mesa Trail contours east around a branch of Charlebois Canyon and climbs north-northwest onto Peters Mesa. Follow the trail as it turns sharply right (east) and climbs over a broad, unnamed saddle on Peters Mesa.

Tip: The trail shown on the U.S.G.S. topo heading northwest toward Squaw Canyon no longer exists.

Descend east into Peters Canyon, and follow the Peters Mesa Trail upstream to the southeast. After 1.1 miles, the trail climbs east away from the wash to the east. Pass over a low saddle and descend almost back to the bed of Peters Canyon. Follow the Peters Mesa Trail as it turns north and climbs to the unnamed saddle between Tortilla Mountain and Horse Ridge. Descend past Kane Spring and continue into Tortilla Canyon. The trail emerges from Tortilla Canyon at the Tortilla Trailhead, 6.7 miles from Charlebois Spring.

POSSIBLE ITINERARY

	Camp	Miles	Elevation Gain
Day 1	Randolph Canyon	9.9	1550
Day 2	La Barge Canyon	9.6	1060
Day 3	Out	6.7	1750

Fish Creek Loop

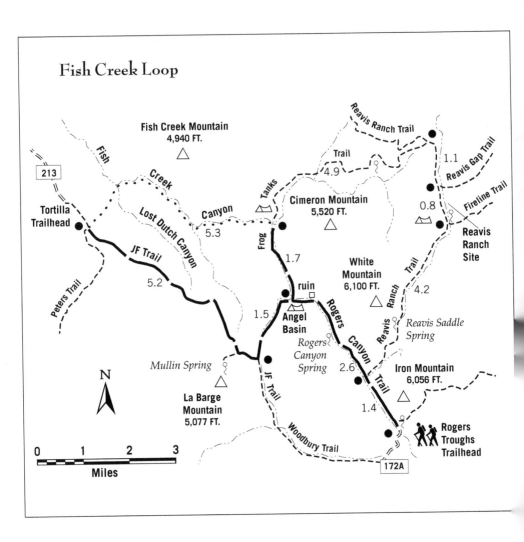

Fish Creek Mountain
4,940 FT.

213

Fish Creek

Lost Dutch Canyon

Canyon

Tortilla
Trailhead

JF Trail

5.2

Peters Trail

Tanks

5.3

Frog

1.7

ruin

1.5

Angel
Basin

Mullin Spring

N

La Barge
Mountain
5,077 FT.

JF Trail

Woodbury Trail

Rogers
Canyon
Spring

0   1   2   3
Miles

Trail
4.9

Cimeron Mountain
5,520 FT.

White
Mountain
6,100 FT.

Rogers

Canyon

Reavis Ranch Trail

Reavis Gap Trail

1.1

0.8

Fireline Trail

Reavis
Ranch
Site

Reavis Ranch Trail

4.2

Reavis Saddle
Spring

2.6

Iron Mountain
6,056 FT.

1.4

Rogers
Troughs
Trailhead

172A

21 Fish Creek Loop

RATINGS (1–10)			MILES	ELEVATION GAIN	DAYS	SHUTTLE MILEAGE
Scenery	Solitude	Difficulty	21.7	3160	3	0
8	6	5	(28.4)	(4260)	(3)	

MAPS Two Bar Mountain, Haunted Canyon, Iron Mountain, Pinyon Mountain U.S.G.S., Superstition Wilderness U.S.F.S.

SEASON September–May.

BEST April–May, October–November.

WATER Seasonal at Rogers Spring, Rogers Canyon Spring, in Fish Creek, Mullin Spring.

PERMITS None.

RULES Maximum group size 15 persons and maximum stay limit of 14 days.

CONTACT Mesa Ranger District, Tonto National Forest, 26 N. MacDonald, P.O. Box 5800, Mesa, Arizona 85211-5800, (480) 610-3300, www.fs.fed.us/r3/tonto.

HIGHLIGHTS The Fish Creek Loop starts with a hike down scenic Rogers Canyon, then loops through a remote, trailless canyon system and along a scenic ridge with views of much of the Superstition Mountains.

PROBLEMS Forest Road 172, the access road, crosses Hewitt Canyon several times, and may be impassable during or after a major storm. The last 0.4 mile of the road requires a high-clearance vehicle.

HOW TO GET THERE From Apache Junction at the east end of the greater Phoenix area, drive 18 miles east on U.S. Highway 60. Turn left (north) on the Queen Creek Road and follow this paved road 1.9 miles. Turn right (east) on dirt Forest Road 357, drive 3.1 miles, and

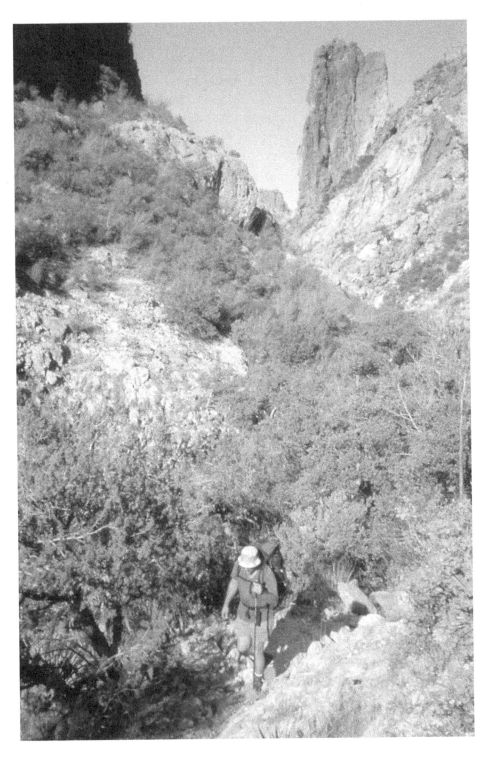

Rogers Canyon

turn left (north) on dirt Forest Road 172. After 12.5 miles, turn right (northeast) on Forest Road 172A. Continue 3.6 miles, staying left on Forest Road 172A at the junction with Forest Road 650, and continue 0.4 mile to the Rogers Troughs Trailhead. The last 0.4 mile requires a high-clearance vehicle.

DESCRIPTION Start the hike on the Reavis Ranch Trail, which descends Rogers Canyon 1.4 miles to the junction with the Rogers Canyon Trail. Optionally, you can remain on the Reavis Ranch Trail to do a longer loop via Reavis Ranch (described later in this section).

Continue the main, shorter loop by turning left (northwest) on the Rogers Canyon Trail and hiking down Rogers Canyon. The scenic canyon gradually deepens as you continue. Where the canyon and trail turn to the west, 2.2 miles from the Reavis Ranch Trail, watch for an unnamed cliff dwelling across the canyon to the right (northwest). This well-preserved ruin is a popular destination, and it has suffered damage from thoughtless visitors. Please leave this and all other ruins and artifacts as you found them. In particular, do not climb on walls or structures. These human dwellings have survived seven or eight hundred years, but can be destroyed in a careless moment. As you continue on the Rogers Canyon Trail, you may find seasonal water in the bed of Rogers Canyon. The canyon opens out into Angel Basin 0.4 mile below the ruin. Angel Basin is a popular scenic campsite and marks the junction with the Frog Tanks Trail.

> **Warning:** Fish Creek, which drains a large area, may be flooding after a major storm. In that case, do not attempt the route down Fish Creek— instead, return the way you came, or consider reversing the Reavis Ranch option.

Turn right (northwest) on the Frog Tanks Trail and continue down Rogers Canyon. Graceful Arizona sycamores and other riparian trees line the canyon bottom. Rogers Canyon ends at Fish Creek, 1.7 miles from Angel Basin. You'll find several small campsites at the confluence and seasonal water in the bed of Fish Creek and Rogers Canyon.

Turn left (west) and hike cross-country down Fish Creek. Though there is no trail, it is easy to walk down the wash—unless it is flooding.

> **Tip:** Pick up water when you find it along Fish Creek. After Fish Creek, you'll follow a dry ridge for 5.2 miles.

▲▲▲ Volcanic Calderas

Much of the central and western Superstition Mountains are the highly eroded remains of a volcanic caldera. Ash and lava flows poured out of volcanic vents and covered large portions of what is now the Superstition Wilderness. As faulting lifted the terrain, erosion carved out deep canyons and cliff-bound mesas and buttes. Remnants of the ancient ash flows can be seen today in the yellow tuff cliffs and the gray rhyolite rocks.

After 5.0 miles of hiking down remote and scenic Fish Creek, Lost Dutch Canyon comes in from the southeast. Leave Fish Creek and hike southwest up an easy slope, staying just west of Lost Dutch Spring. As you come out onto the crest of a ridge that trends southeast, you'll intercept the JF Trail about a mile southeast of its beginning at the Tortilla Ranch Trailhead, 1.1 miles after leaving Fish Creek.

Tip: Watch carefully for the trail, which is faint and easily confused by cattle trails.

Turn left (southeast) on the JF Trail. The trail climbs along the top of the nameless ridge above Lost Dutch Canyon. The view of the central and western Superstition Mountains unfolds as you continue. As you approach seasonal Clover Spring, the JF Trail stays on the west slopes of the ridge for 1.3 miles. After you pass through a saddle near the head of Lost Dutch Canyon, the trail rejoins the ridge crest above the head of Goat Canyon. For 2.0 miles the high ridge provides the best views of the trip. Follow the JF Trail southeast through the saddle dividing Goat Canyon from Tortilla Creek. As the trail turns east, you'll pass the spur trail to Mullin Spring, located in a side canyon about 0.5 mile west. Continue east on the JF Trail and climb to another saddle at the head of Tortilla Creek. The nameless pass, 5.2 miles from where you intercepted the JF Trail, is the junction with the Rogers Canyon Trail.

Turn left (north) and follow the Rogers Canyon Trail over another nameless saddle. This 4600-foot pass is the high point of the trip. Descend to the north-northeast, following an unnamed tributary of Rogers Canyon. After 1.5 miles, you'll meet the Frog Tanks Trail at Angel Basin, closing the loop. Stay right (east) on the Rogers Canyon Trail and hike 4.0 miles to the Rogers Troughs Trailhead.

	Camp	Miles	Elevation Gain
Day 1	Fish Creek	5.7	0
Day 2	Angel Basin	12.0	2040
Day 3	Out	4.0	1120

REAVIS RANCH OPTIONAL EXTENDED LOOP From the junction of the Reavis Ranch Trail and the Rogers Canyon Trail, turn right (northeast) and follow the Reavis Ranch Trail past the Reavis Ranch site. For details on this trail, see the Campaign Creek Loop. North of the old ranch site, stay left on the Reavis Ranch Trail, and follow it 1.1 miles out of Reavis Creek to the first of several broad saddles. Turn left (southwest) on the Frog Tanks Trail and descend into the headwaters of Paradise Canyon, a tributary of Fish Creek. Soon you'll pass Plow Saddle Springs, marked by a concrete watering trough. If the trough is dry, follow the drainage above the trail to the actual springs.

Continue the descent on the Frog Tanks Trail along a bench north of Paradise Creek. The trail reaches the confluence of Paradise and Fish creeks 3.1 miles from the Reavis Ranch Trail. Follow the Frog Tanks Trail across Fish Creek and downstream to the west and south. The U.S.G.S. topographic map shows the trail staying in the bed down to the mouth of Rough Canyon, but actually it climbs to the map location of Frog Spring. The only sign of this spring is a gravel-filled cement trough, but there may be water in wet years.

Finally, the trail crosses a flat-topped ridge at the 3600-foot contour, and then descends steeply to Fish Creek at the mouth of Rogers Canyon, where you join the main loop hike. You'll find camping for small groups here.

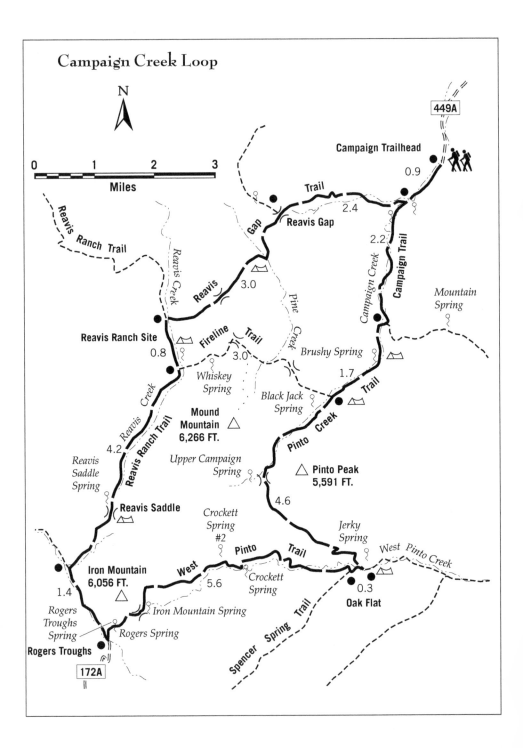

Campaign Creek Loop

N

0 1 2 3
Miles

449A

Campaign Trailhead

0.9

Reavis Ranch Trail

Reavis Creek

Gap

Reavis Trail Reavis Gap

2.4

2.2

Campaign Creek

Campaign Trail

3.0

Pine Creek

Mountain Spring

Reavis Ranch Site

0.8

Fireline Trail

3.0

Reavis Creek

Brushy Spring

1.7

Whiskey Spring

Black Jack Spring

Pinto Creek Trail

Mound Mountain 6,266 FT. △

4.2

Reavis Ranch Trail

Upper Campaign Spring

△ Pinto Peak 5,591 FT.

Reavis Saddle Spring

Reavis Saddle

Crockett Spring #2

4.6

Jerky Spring

West Pinto Creek

West Pinto Trail

1.4

Iron Mountain 6,056 FT. △

West

5.6

Crockett Spring

0.3

Oak Flat

Rogers Troughs Spring

Iron Mountain Spring

Rogers Spring

Spencer Spring Trail

Rogers Troughs

172A

22   Campaign Creek Loop

RATINGS (1–10)			MILES	ELEVATION GAIN	DAYS	SHUTTLE MILEAGE
Scenery	Solitude	Difficulty	29.9	5820	3	0
7	7	5	(14.9)	(2960)	(2)	

MAPS Two Bar Mountain, Haunted Canyon, Iron Mountain, Pinyon Mountain U.S.G.S., Superstition Wilderness U.S.F.S.

SEASON September–May.

BEST October–November, April–May.

WATER Campaign Creek, seasonal at Brushy Spring, Black Jack Spring, Crockett Spring, Iron Mountain Spring, Rogers Spring, Reavis Saddle Spring, Reavis Creek, Pine Creek, Walnut Spring.

PERMITS None.

RULES Maximum group size 15 persons and maximum stay limit of 14 days.

CONTACT Mesa Ranger District, Tonto National Forest, 26 N. MacDonald, P.O. Box 5800, Mesa, Arizona 85211-5800, (480) 610-3300, www.fs.fed.us/r3/tonto.

HIGHLIGHTS The Campaign Creek Loop hike follows trails in the eastern Superstition Mountains, the highest section of the range. Hikers familiar with the Sonoran desert in the western Superstition Mountains will be surprised to find stands of ponderosa pine tucked away in the eastern section. Other attractions include a historic ranch site and an optional side hike to Mound Mountain, the highest summit in the Superstition Mountains.

PROBLEMS The road to the Campaign Trailhead receives little maintenance, and may be impassable during or after a major storm.

HOW TO GET THERE Starting from Apache Junction at the east side of the Phoenix metro area, drive 48.6 miles east on Arizona 88 (20 miles of which is all-weather gravel). Turn right on Forest Road 449, the Campaign Creek Road, a maintained dirt road, and drive 1.9 miles. Turn left at a fork onto Forest Road 449A. This road crosses Campaign Creek several times and receives little maintenance. It may be impassable during and after a major storm. Drive 5.2 miles on Forest Road 449A to the Campaign Trailhead. The trailhead is on private land—please park in the signed trailhead parking. Camping is not allowed at the trailhead.

Tip: The first section of the trail passes through the grounds of the Reavis Mountain School (formerly the Upper Horrell Ranch). Please respect private property and stay on the trail.

DESCRIPTION Follow the Campaign Trail southwest through the school and up Campaign Creek. This section of Campaign Creek has a perennial stream, a delight in this otherwise dry desert grassland. The Reavis Gap Trail comes in from the right 0.9 mile from the Campaign Trailhead. Stay right on the Campaign Trail and continue south along Campaign Creek. Just 0.6 mile beyond the trail junction, the trail climbs over a saddle to avoid a difficult section of the canyon bottom. The Campaign Creek Trail descends back to the creek where it remains. Arizona sycamore trees grace the canyon bottom, a contrast to the dull green of the brushy canyon walls. When you've hiked 2.2 miles from the Reavis Gap Trail junction, the Campaign Trail ends at the Pinto Creek Trail. Turn right (south) and follow the Pinto Creek Trail up Campaign Creek. You'll find plenty of campsites, though the creek may be dry. Brushy Spring has water except in dry years. Just 1.7 miles from the Campaign Trail, you'll meet the Fireline Trail junction, which offers a scenic shortcut that shortens the trip to an over-night visit.

Continue the main loop on the Pinto Creek Trail southwest up Campaign Creek. Ponderosa pines start to appear as you approach the head of Campaign Creek. Climb southwest on the Pinto Creek Trail to a scenic saddle overlooking West Pinto Creek. Descend south and southeast from the saddle onto a ridge, and follow the trail down to Oak Flat, 4.6 miles from the Fireline Trail junction. You'll find plenty of campsites at Oak Flat, and possibly water in the bed of West

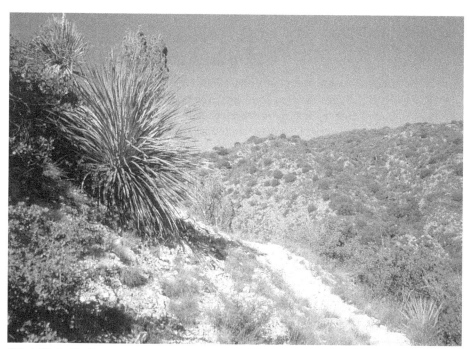
West Pinto Trail

Pinto Creek. If not, check Jerky Spring, 0.7 mile up the Cuff Button Trail to the north of Oak Flat.

Turn right (west) on the West Pinto Trail and hike up West Pinto Creek. The Spencer Spring Trail junction is at the west edge of Oak Flat. Stay right (west) and continue on the West Pinto Trail up West Pinto Creek. The trail climbs along the south side of West Pinto Creek for 0.8 mile, then descends to cross the creek. The West Pinto Trail stays on the north side of the canyon for 1.3 miles, descends to the bed, and follows it upstream. Look for seasonal water where the U.S.F.S. wilderness map shows Crockett Spring. The U.S.F.S. Wilderness map also shows a spur trail going north to Crockett Spring #2, but this trail may be overgrown and hard to find. Follow the West Pinto Trail along West Pinto Creek for 0.7 mile, where it veers away from the creek and up a steep ridge. This ridge is brushy and the trail may be overgrown. When the West Pinto Trail reaches the east slopes of Iron Mountain, it turns south and descends to pass Iron Mountain Spring. Follow the trail west over the south ridge of Iron Mountain and descend the grassy slopes into Rogers Canyon. After the West

♨ Reavis Ranch

An active cattle ranch until the 1960s, Reavis Ranch was then sold to the U.S. Forest Service. The Forest Service intended to preserve the old ranch house as a historic structure, but vandals ruined the building. Finally, a careless camper started a fire that consumed the ranch building, and the U.S. Forest Service and volunteers cleaned up the remains. One notable remnant of the ranching days remains—the apple orchard, found downstream from the ranch site. Access to the ranch was via a long and winding dirt road from Arizona Highway 88. As you hike north of the ranch on the Reavis Ranch Trail, you're following the old road. After the U.S. Forest Service acquired the ranch, the old road was added to the Superstition Wilderness and closed to motorized travel.

Pinto Trail passes Rogers Spring, it ends at the junction with the Reavis Ranch Trail, 5.6 miles from Oak Flat.

Turn right (northwest) and follow the Reavis Ranch Trail northwest down Rogers Canyon. Just 1.4 miles from the West Pinto Trail, you'll meet the Rogers Canyon Trail. Turn right (northeast) and follow the Reavis Ranch Trail up Grave Canyon. Climb steadily for 1.3 miles to reach broad Reavis Saddle. You'll find a few small campsites in this area, but the only water source is unreliable Reavis Saddle Spring. Continue north on the Reavis Ranch Trail, which gently descends the headwaters of Reavis Creek through pinyon pine and juniper woodland and occasional ponderosa pine. You'll pass the Fireline Trail junction 4.2 miles from the Rogers Canyon Trail junction. You can usually find water in Reavis Creek north of the Fireline Trail. The site of Reavis Ranch is 0.4 mile north of the Fireline Trail in a series of meadows along Reavis Valley. You'll find plenty of campsites along the meadows.

Follow the Reavis Ranch Trail north 0.5 mile along the west side of the old apple orchard to the junction with the Reavis Gap Trail. Turn right (east) on the Reavis Gap Trail, cross Reavis Creek, and climb east out of the valley over a nameless saddle next to a small knob. Follow the Reavis Gap Trail as it descends gently to cross Pine Creek. You'll find campsites at Pine Creek, and plenty of water in wet years. After crossing the creek, the trail climbs gradually to Reavis Gap, a broad, grassy saddle overlooking Campaign Creek. At the junction with the Two Bar Ridge Trail, stay right (east) on the Reavis

Gap Trail and descend 2.4 miles to the Campaign Trail. Turn left (north) and hike 0.9 mile to the Campaign Trailhead.

POSSIBLE ITINERARY

	Camp	Miles	Elevation Gain
Day 1	Oak Flat	9.4	2100
Day 2	Reavis Ranch	11.6	2940
Day 3	Out	6.7	780

FIRELINE TRAIL OPTIONAL SHORTCUT The Fireline Trail climbs steeply west to a pass overlooking the headwaters of Pine Creek and descends to the creek. Follow the Fireline Trail southwest up Pine Creek, then northwest up a nameless tributary. Cross a nameless saddle, then continue past Whiskey Spring to the end of the Fireline Trail at the junction with the Reavis Ranch Trail, 3.0 miles from the Pinto Peak Trail. Turn right (north) on the Reavis Ranch Trail to join the main loop.

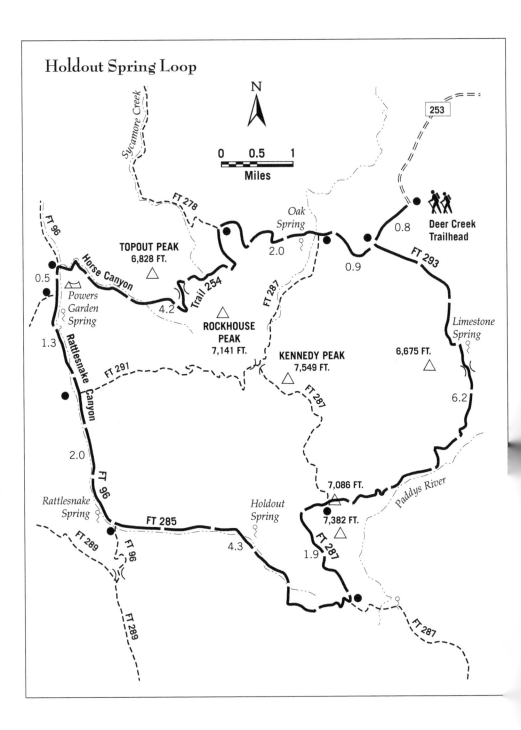

Holdout Spring Loop

N

0   0.5   1
Miles

253

Sycamore Creek

FT 278

FT 96

*Oak
Spring*

0.8

**Deer Creek
Trailhead**

TOPOUT PEAK
6,828 FT.

2.0

0.9

FT 293

Horse Canyon

0.5

*Powers
Garden
Spring*

Trail 254

4.2

FT 287

*Limestone
Spring*

1.3

Rattlesnake Canyon

**ROCKHOUSE
PEAK**
7,141 FT.

KENNEDY PEAK
7,549 FT.

6,675 FT.

6.2

FT 291

FT 287

2.0

FT 96

7,086 FT.

Paddys River

*Rattlesnake
Spring*

*Holdout
Spring*

FT 285

7,382 FT.

FT 289

FT 96

4.3

1.9

FT 287

FT 289

FT 287

23   Holdout Spring Loop

RATINGS (1–10)			MILES	ELEVATION GAIN	DAYS	SHUTTLE MILEAGE
Scenery	Solitude	Difficulty	25.0	5520	3	0
7	9	6				

MAPS Kennedy Peak U.S.G.S.

SEASON September–November, March–May.

BEST October–November, April.

WATER Seasonal at Limestone Spring, Holdout Spring, Rattlesnake Spring, and Powers Garden Spring,

PERMITS None.

RULES None.

CONTACT Safford Ranger District, Coronado National Forest, PO Box 709, Safford, Arizona 85548-0709, (520) 428-4150, www.fs.fed.us/ r3/coronado.

HIGHLIGHTS If you want to hike the trail less traveled, the Galiuro Mountains are the place. One of southern Arizona's less known sky islands, this rugged range is attractive not only because of its remoteness, but also because of its interesting history.

PROBLEMS Trails in the Galiuro Mountains receive little maintenance and sections may be brushy and overgrown. You should carry the U.S.G.S. topographic maps, which accurately show the trails on the Holdout Spring Loop. Water is scarce, especially at the start, so all party members should have enough water capacity for a dry camp.

HOW TO GET THERE From Safford, drive 15.3 miles west on U.S. 70 and turn left (southwest) on Klondyke Road. Drive 24.6 miles on this maintained dirt road and turn left (northwest) on Aravaipa Road, which is also maintained dirt. Drive 4.4 miles and turn right on Deer

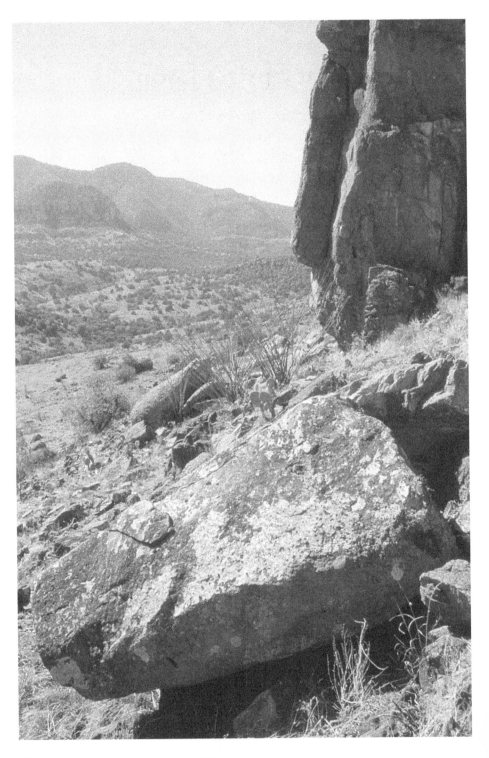

Near Deer Creek, Galiuro Mountains

Creek Road (Forest Road 253). Follow this rough dirt road 6.6 miles to its end at the Deer Creek Trailhead.

DESCRIPTION Hike 0.8 mile southwest on Forest Trail 254 to the junction of Forest Trails 254 and 293. Turn left (southeast) on Forest Trail 293 to start the loop. Follow Forest Trail 293 south past Deer Creek Ranch through juniper woodland. You'll pass Limestone Spring as the trail climbs the headwaters of Gardner Creek to an unnamed pass, 2.4 miles from Forest Trail 254.

Tip: Keep your water containers topped up, and be prepared for a dry camp.

Follow Forest Trail 293 south across an unnamed canyon, over a ridge, and southwest down to Paddys River, which is 1.8 miles from the unnamed pass. Paddys River is actually a seasonal creek, and you may not find water during dry periods. The trail stays near the river for 0.7 mile, and this is your first opportunity to camp.

Tip: Ahead, the trail stays on dry ridges for 5.5 miles before reaching the next water source at Holdout Spring.

Follow Forest Trail 293 as it climbs steeply onto the ridge to the west. You'll reach the crest and the junction of Forest Trails 287 and 293 at Peak 7086, 1.2 miles from Paddys River. Turn left (west) on Forest Trail 287 and follow the trail along the ridge into a saddle. Turn south and climb over Peak 7382 to the junction of Forest Trails 287 and 285, 1.9 miles from Peak 7086.

Tip: There is an unnamed spring 0.7 mile east on Forest Trail 287, at the head of Paddys River.

Turn right on Forest Trail 285 and descend the brushy ridge west 1.0 mile to an unnamed saddle. Turn north and follow the trail as it descends into the headwaters of Rattlesnake Canyon and turns northwest along the canyon bottom. When you've hiked 2.2 miles from the junction of Forest Trails 287 and 285, Rattlesnake Canyon turns west and a 0.2-mile spur trail on the right (northeast) leads to Holdout Spring and cave. Continue 2.1 miles west along Rattlesnake Canyon to the junction of Forest Trails 285 and 96. Optionally, you can do an 0.9-mile side hike south to a viewpoint.

To continue the main loop turn right (northwest) on Forest Trail 96. After 0.3 mile, you'll pass Rattlesnake Spring, which is on the right side of Rattlesnake Canyon just before canyon turns north.

Powers Garden

Powers Garden is the site of a ranch that was established by the Powers brothers around 1900. The two brothers were active with mining and ranching throughout the central Galiuro Mountains, and remnants of their work can be seen up and down Rattlesnake Canyon. There used to be a wagon road up Rattlesnake Canyon from the north, but it has reverted to a foot trail and the entire area has been added to the Galiuro Wilderness. The Powers brothers were accused of avoiding the draft during World War I, and when the sheriff came to arrest them, they fled up Rattlesnake Canyon.

Follow Forest Trail 96 north past the mouth of Douglas Canyon to the junction of Forest Trails 291 and 96 at the mouth of Corral Canyon, 2.0 miles from Forest Trail 285. Hike 1.3 miles along Rattlesnake Canyon to another trail junction and the gorgeous, pine-rimmed meadow at Powers Garden. You'll find plenty of campsites, and water at Powers Garden Spring just south of the old ranch buildings.

Hike north 0.5 mile along Rattlesnake Canyon to the junction of Forest Trails 96 and 254. Turn right (east) and follow Forest Trail 254 through an S-turn in Horse Canyon. The trail climbs southeast up the canyon to a fork. Follow Forest Trail 254 up the left (north) fork and up a switchback to Topout Divide. This low point on the ridge between Rockhouse and Topout Peaks is 2.4 miles from Rattlesnake Canyon. Continue east on Forest Trail 254 east and contour around the headwaters of Sycamore Creek.

Follow the trail north onto the ridge between Oak Creek and Sycamore Creek and to the junction of Forest Trails 278 and 254, 1.8 miles from Topout Divide. Descend east on Forest Trail 254 across two unnamed tributaries of Oak Creek and cross Oak Creek at the junction of Forest Trails 287 and 254. Stay on Forest Trail 254 0.9 mile to the top of the ridge at the head of Deer Creek and the junction of Forest Trails 254 and 293. Hike 0.8 mile northeast on Forest Trail 254 to the Deer Creek Trailhead.

	Camp	Miles	Elevation Gain
Day 1	Upper Paddys River	5.3	1500
Day 2	Powers Garden	11.3	2060
Day 3	Out	8.4	1960

Tip: The following itinerary assumes that you have done the approach drive in the morning and will have a half-day left to hike on the first day. You may want to add another day to avoid the long hike on Day 2.

KIELBURG CANYON OPTIONAL SIDE HIKE From the junction of Forest Trails 285 and 96, turn left (south) and hike 0.9 mile to the unnamed saddle at the head of Kielburg Canyon. This spot offers great views of the interior of the Galiuro Wilderness.

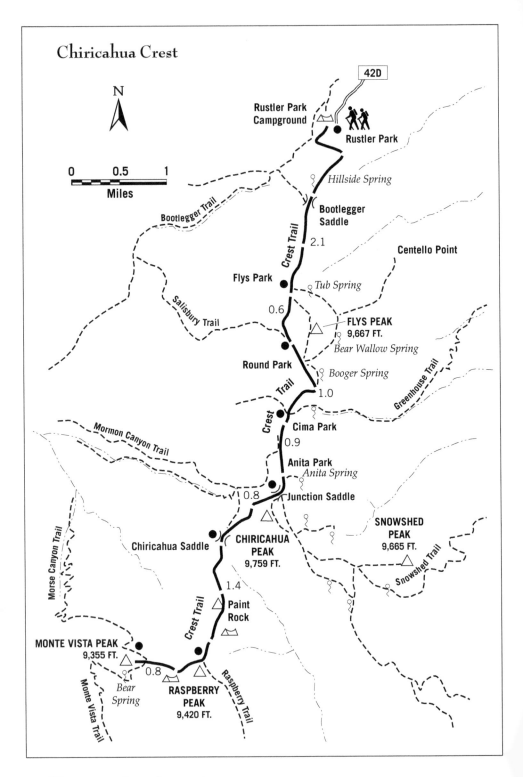

Chiricahua Crest

N

0   0.5   1
Miles

42D

Rustler Park
Campground

Rustler Park

Hillside Spring

Bootlegger Trail

Bootlegger
Saddle
2.1

Crest Trail

Centello Point

Flys Park

Tub Spring

0.6

Salisbury Trail

FLYS PEAK
9,667 FT.

Bear Wallow Spring

Round Park

Booger Spring

Greenhouse Trail

Crest Trail

1.0

Cima Park

Mormon Canyon Trail

0.9

Anita Park
Anita Spring

Crest Trail

0.8

Junction Saddle

**SNOWSHED
PEAK**
9,665 FT.

Morse Canyon Trail

Chiricahua Saddle

**CHIRICAHUA
PEAK**
9,759 FT.

Snowshed Trail

1.4

Paint
Rock

MONTE VISTA PEAK
9,355 FT.

Crest Trail

Raspberry Trail

0.8

*Bear
Spring*

Monte Vista Trail

**RASPBERRY
PEAK**
9,420 FT.

24 Chiricahua Crest

RATINGS (1–10)			MILES	ELEVATION GAIN	DAYS	SHUTTLE MILEAGE
Scenery	Solitude	Difficulty	15.2	1890	2	0
8	3	3				

MAPS Rustler Park, Chiricahua Peak U.S.G.S.

SEASON May–November.

BEST June–October.

WATER Seasonal at Tub, Booger, Anita, and Bear Springs. You'll find several other springs near the route.

PERMITS None.

RULES None

CONTACT Douglas Ranger District, Coronado National Forest, 3081 North Leslie Canyon Road, Douglas, Arizona 85607, (520) 364-3468, www.fs.fed.us/r3/coronado.

HIGHLIGHTS This out-and-back hike takes you along the scenic crest of the Chiricahua Mountains, another of southern Arizona's sky island ranges. The trail wanders through cool Douglas-fir and quaking aspen forest, and passes the highest peaks of the range enroute to Monte Vista Peak at the south end of the range. This 9355-foot summit rewards you with sweeping views of southeast Arizona and northern Mexico.

PROBLEMS Water is scarce since the trail stays on ridges. In the spring you may encounter lingering snowdrifts. Black bears are common and have been known to raid campsites for food. Hang your food or use a bear-proof backpacker's food container.

Warning: All of the springs on this hike are seasonal. Carry enough water for a dry camp.

HOW TO GET THERE Starting from Willcox on Interstate 10, drive east on Arizona 186 34 miles and turn left on Arizona 181. Drive 3.0 miles and turn left on graded dirt Pinery Canyon Road (Forest Road 42). Drive 12.0 miles to Onion Saddle and turn right on the Rustler Park Road (Forest Road 42D). Drive 3.0 miles south to Rustler Park Trailhead at Rustler Park Campground.

DESCRIPTION Follow the Crest Trail 0.2 mile southwest to the junction with the Buena Vista Peak Trail. Stay left (south) on the Crest Trail and contour southeast along the east side of the crest. Follow the trail to Bootlegger Saddle and the junction with the Bootlegger Trail. Stay left (south) on the Crest Trail as it climbs to avoid steep terrain on the west side of the crest, reaching 9200 feet before descending to a saddle at Flys Park, 2.1 miles from the trailhead. Tub Spring lies 0.2 mile east on a spur trail.

Follow the Crest Trail 0.6 mile south to the junction with the Salisbury Trail. Stay left (south) on the Crest Trail as it contours west of the crest and continues south 0.3 mile to Round Park, where a spur trail goes 0.2 mile east to Booger Spring. Several of the parks near the start of the hike are popular campsites.

> **Tip:** *Avoid the crowds by carrying enough water for a dry camp, and plan to camp south of Chiricahua Peak.*

Continue the main hike on the Crest Trail and contour east of the crest 0.7 mile to Cima Park and the junction with the Greenhouse Trail. Hike 0.8 mile south on the Crest Trail along the west side of the crest to Anita Park, where yet another spur trail leads 0.2 mile east to Anita Spring.

⚘ Parks

Used locally in southeast Arizona and southwest New Mexico to refer to meadows, the term "park" is common on maps of the region. Most parks were probably created by forest fires. Naturally occurring fires normally burn at low intensity and do not kill the trees, but there are often hot spots where conditions cause a fire to crown. Such hot fires kill the trees, creating small meadows. Along the Chiricahua Crest, quaking aspen is the first tree to invade meadows. The aspens provide shade for less sun-tolerant trees such as Douglas-fir. Eventually fir or pine crowds out the short-lived aspen, returning the forest to its prefire condition over a span of 500 years or more.

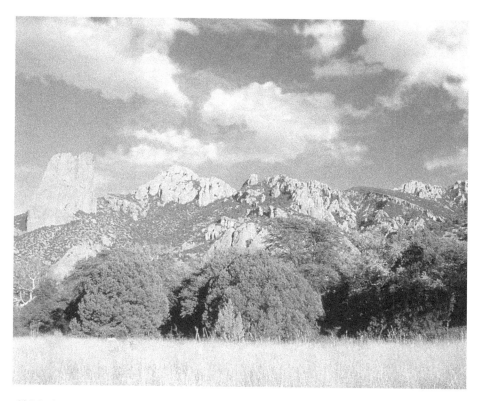

Chiricahua Mountains

Tip: *This is the last spring along the trail, so make sure you have enough water for a dry camp.*

Just 0.1 mile farther south the Crest Trail meets the Snowshed Trail at Junction Saddle. Turn right (southwest) on the Crest Trail and hike 0.8 mile to Chiricahua Saddle.

Hike south on the Crest Trail, which stays on the crest except where it passes Paint Rock on the east. After 1.4 miles you'll meet the Raspberry Trail. Turn right and follow the Crest Trail 0.8 mile past Raspberry Peak to Monte Vista Peak.

Tip: *Monte Vista Peak is closed to camping, so look for a campsite between Chricahua Saddle and the unnamed saddle east of Monte Vista Peak.*

The fire lookout tower on Monte Vista Peak is staffed during the summer fire season. Ask permission before climbing the tower. In

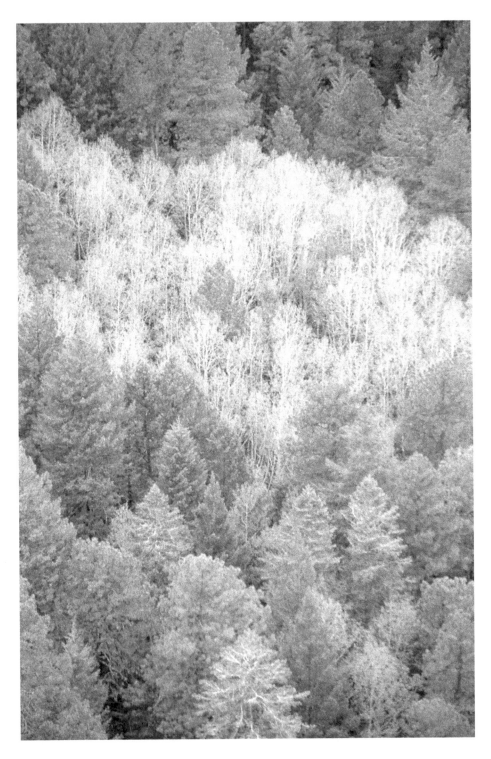

Aspens in Chiricahua Mountains

contrast to heavily forested Chiricahua Peak, Monte Vista Peak is bald and offers great views of the southern Chiricahua Mountains, southeast Arizona, and northern Sonora, Mexico. Return to the trailhead the way you came.

POSSIBLE ITINERARY

	Camp	Miles	Elevation Gain
Day 1	Raspberry Peak	8.4	1380
Day 2	Out	6.6	510

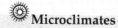 **Microclimates**

Plant and animal communities are extremely sensitive to their environment. As you hike the Crest Trail, notice how the forest changes from Douglas-fir to pine and back as the trail traverse north- and south-facing slopes. Just a slight change in aspect (the direction the slope faces) causes a change in the local climate. South-facing slopes receive more heat from the sun and have a higher evaporation rate, while north slopes are cooler and moister. Heat-tolerant trees such as ponderosa and Apache pine favor south aspects, while Douglas-fir and quaking aspen prefer north slopes.

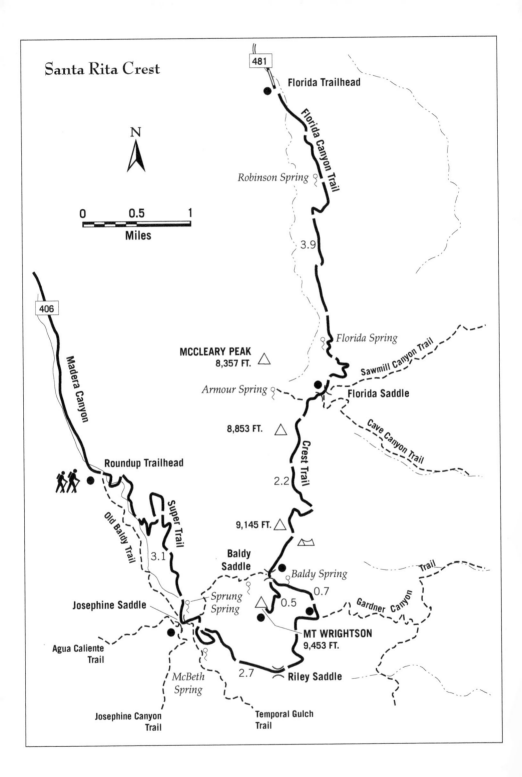

Santa Rita Crest

481

Florida Trailhead

Florida Canyon Trail

N

0   0.5   1
Miles

Robinson Spring

3.9

Florida Spring

Sawmill Canyon Trail

406

Madera Canyon

MCCLEARY PEAK
8,357 FT.

Armour Spring

Florida Saddle

8,853 FT.

Cave Canyon Trail

Roundup Trailhead

Crest Trail

2.2

Super Trail

9,145 FT.

Old Baldy Trail

3.1

Baldy
Saddle

Baldy Spring

Trail

0.7

Josephine Saddle

Sprung
Spring

0.5

Gardner Canyon

Agua Caliente
Trail

MT WRIGHTSON
9,453 FT.

McBeth
Spring

2.7

Riley Saddle

Josephine Canyon
Trail

Temporal Gulch
Trail

25 Santa Rita Crest

RATINGS (1–10)			MILES	ELEVATION GAIN	DAYS	SHUTTLE MILEAGE
Scenery	Solitude	Difficulty	13.3	4030	2	9.0
8	3	4				

MAPS Mount Wrightson U.S.G.S.

SEASON April–November.

BEST May–October.

WATER Madera Creek, and seasonally at Sprung, Baldy, Armour, Florida, and Robinson Springs.

PERMITS None.

RULES None.

CONTACT Nogales Ranger District, Coronado National Forest, 303 Old Tucson Road, Nogales, Arizona 85621, (520) 281-2296, www.fs.fed.us/r3/coronado.

HIGHLIGHTS The one-way Santa Rita Crest hike starts along Madera Canyon, which features a flowing stream and is a world-famous birding site. A short spur trail can be done as a side trip to Mount Wrightson, the 9453-foot summit of the Santa Rita Mountains. The remainder of the trip follows the scenic Santa Rita Crest Trail northward. Cliffs and rock outcrops along the crest of the Santa Rita Mountains break up the alpine forest and provide several views of the grassy valleys and other sky island ranges of southeast Arizona and northern Mexico.

PROBLEMS Because you'll be climbing over 4000 feet, the weather is cooler on the crest than at the trailheads. In the summer, this is a delight, but keep a wary eye on the weather during spring and late fall. Winter snowstorms can move in suddenly, and much of the route is exposed to the weather. From May through September the weather is hot at lower elevations; carry plenty of water. Thunderstorms and lightning are common from July through mid September.

HOW TO GET THERE To reach the end trailhead from Tucson, drive 24 miles south on Interstate 19, and exit at the town of Continental. Drive east through Continental, and continue 8.1 miles on paved Madera Canyon Road (Forest Road 62). At the junction with dirt Forest Road 62 continue straight (east). After 0.3 mile, turn right (south) on Forest Road 62A, and continue 2.9 miles to the Florida Trailhead at the end of the road.

To reach the start trailhead, retrace your route to the Madera Canyon Road, turn left (south), and drive 5.8 miles to the end of the road at the Roundup Trailhead.

Tip: The best direction to do this hike is as described, from south to north, because the Roundup Trailhead is 1100 feet higher than the Florida Trailhead.

DESCRIPTION Hike up Madera Canyon on the well-named Super Trail, which climbs at a steady grade. This trail was built to replace the shorter, steeper Old Baldy Trail, which is still shown on the maps. After 1.0 mile, the Super Trail switchbacks above Madera Creek, eventually climbing around a small hill and passing through a low saddle. Continue the steady climb along the east side of Madera Canyon past Sprung Spring to Josephine Saddle, 3.1 miles from the Roundup Trailhead.

Tip: Pick up water from Sprung Spring for a dry camp. Although you'll pass one more spring on the Super Trail, it's a good idea not to depend on a single source.

Four trails branch off in or near this saddle, but stay on the Super Trail south along the east slopes of Mount Wrightson. The trail uses a long switchback to gain altitude and heads out along the southwest slopes of the peak. Pass through Riley Saddle, a dip in the ridge connecting Mount Wrightson and Josephine Peak, and follow the Super Trail northeast to the junction with the Gardner Canyon Trail, 2.7 miles from Josephine Saddle. Another 0.7 mile of steady ascent leads past Baldy Spring to Baldy Saddle and the junction of the Super Trail, old Baldy Trail, and Santa Rita Crest Trail. Optionally, you can climb Mount Wrightson.

Continue the main hike north on the Santa Rita Crest Trail. You'll find the best campsites along the first 0.5 mile of the Crest Trail, where the trail stays near the actual crest.

Warning: *Do not underestimate the weather along the crest of the range, especially during late fall or winter. Campers have died on this mountain after being caught in a winter snow storm. Also, be alert for afternoon thunderstorms from July through mid-September. If thunderstorm activity is high, you may not want to camp along the crest.*

When you are 0.6 mile from Baldy Saddle, the Santa Rita Crest Trail descends onto the east slope of the range and contours north through an unnamed saddle. Follow the Crest Trail as it descends in earnest past the 0.3-mile spur trail to Armour Spring to end at Florida Saddle, 2.2 miles from Baldy Saddle. Three additional trails leave this saddle. Turn left (north) on the Florida Canyon Trail and descend rapidly into Florida Canyon. Florida Spring is 1.0 mile from Florida Saddle, and after this water source the trail descends the east side of the canyon. The Florida Canyon Trail descends along a ridge, skirts the head of a small side canyon, and passes just east of Robinson Spring. A final mile brings you to the Florida Trailhead.

POSSIBLE ITINERARY

	Camp	Miles	Elevation Gain
Day 1	North of Baldy Saddle	7.6	4030
Day 2	Out	5.7	0

MOUNT WRIGHTSON OPTIONAL SIDE TRIP At the junction of the Super Trail, old Baldy Trail, and Santa Rita Crest Trail, turn left (south) on the Old Baldy Trail. This rocky trail climbs the north and east sides of the peak, leading to the summit in just 0.5 mile. As you would expect, views from the bald summit are impressive. Mexico, just 25 miles distant, spreads out across the southern horizon. To the west, the Tumacacori and Baboquivari Mountains form the skyline, while the massive bulk of the Rincon and Santa Catalina Mountains lies to the north, near Tucson. To the southeast, the lush grasslands of the Sonoita Valley lie at your feet, and beyond you can see the Patagonia and Huachuca Mountains.

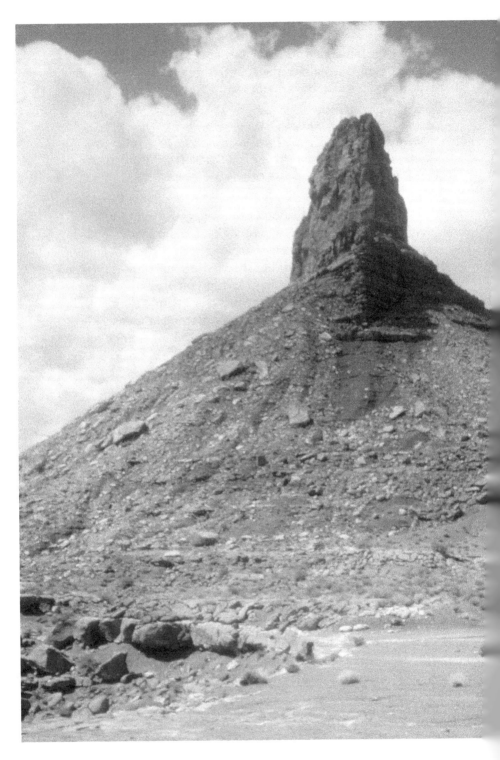

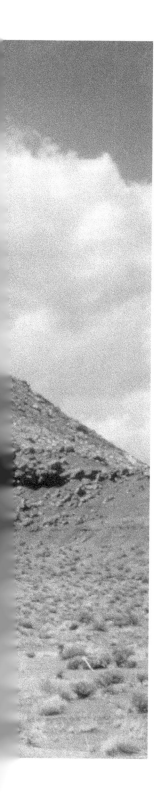

Other Backpacking
Trips

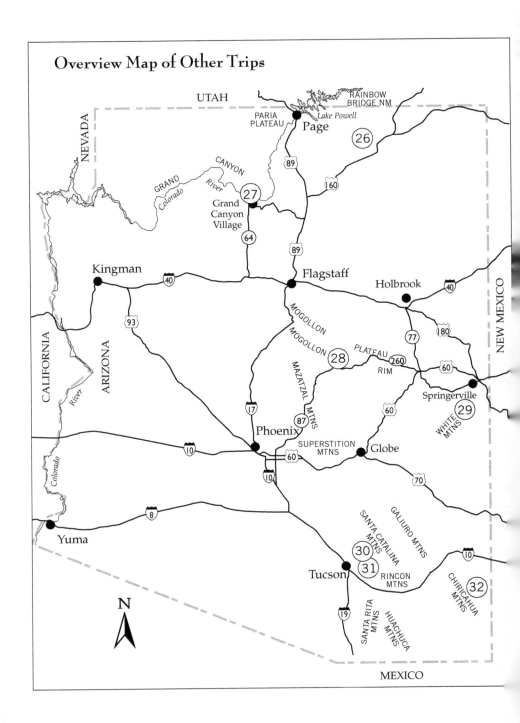

Overview Map of Other Trips

UTAH

NEVADA

RAINBOW
BRIDGE NM

PARIA
PLATEAU

Lake Powell

Page

26

89

160

GRAND CANYON

Colorado River

27

Grand
Canyon
Village

64

89

Kingman

40

93

CALIFORNIA

ARIZONA

Colorado River

Flagstaff

Holbrook

40

NEW MEXICO

MOGOLLON

MOGOLLON

28

PLATEAU

RIM

77

180

260

60

MAZATZAL MTNS

17

60

Springerville

29

WHITE MTNS

Phoenix

87

SUPERSTITION MTNS

Globe

60

10

60

70

8

10

Yuma

SANTA CATALINA MTNS

GALIURO MTNS

30

31

10

Tucson

RINCON MTNS

CHIRICAHUA MTNS

32

19

SANTA RITA MTNS

HUACHUCA MTNS

N

MEXICO

26   Keet Seel

RATINGS (1–10)			MILES	DAYS
Scenery	Solitude	Difficulty	16.6	2
9	2	4		

MAPS Betatakin Ruin, Keet Seel Ruin, Tall Mountain, Marsh Pass U.S.G.S.

SEASON Memorial Day through Labor Day.

BEST May.

HIGHLIGHTS Keet Seel is one of the largest and best preserved Anasazi ruins in the Southwest, and it is protected in a division of Navajo National Monument. The overnight, out-and-back hike to the ruin is a popular, classic desert hike through towering sandstone canyons.

PROBLEMS The trail to Keet Seel is only open when Park Service rangers staff the Keet Seel area. A permit must be obtained from the Visitor Center. The trail and the national monument units are on Navajo Reservation land, and hikers must stay on the trail. Camping is allowed only in the campground at Keet Seel.

HOW TO GET THERE From Flagstaff, drive north on U.S. 89 and northeast on U.S. 160, and turn left on Arizona 564. Continue to the end of the road at the Navajo National Monument Visitor Center.

DESCRIPTION The Keet Seel Trail descends into Betatakin Canyon, named after another Anasazi ruin and crosses Tsegi Canyon and heads up Dowozhiebito and Keet Seel Canyons to Keet Seel Ruin. The main difficulty of the hike is deep sand along the trail.

27 Boucher Trail to Bright Angel Trail

RATINGS (1–10)			MILES	DAYS
Scenery	Solitude	Difficulty	26.9	5
10	5	6		

MAPS Grand Canyon, Piute Point U.S.G.S.

SEASON Mid September–May.

BEST October–November, March–April.

HIGHLIGHTS The Boucher to Bright Angel hike is a classic Grand Canyon backpack trip from the south rim. Grand Canyon offers enough great backpack trips to last a lifetime, but there had to be room in this book for other Arizona hikes! Boucher, Hermit, and Monument Creeks flow year–round and they provide excellent side hikes to the Colorado River. During the summer half of the year, a free shuttle runs from the Bright Angel Trailhead in Grand Canyon Village to the Hermit Trailhead at Hermits Rest, so you can do this without a shuttle vehicle, or any vehicle at all. Public transportation (air, bus, and rail) is available to Grand Canyon Village.

PROBLEMS Like all Grand Canyon backpack trips, this one involves a great deal of elevation loss and gain. The canyon is much warmer than the rim, which is a benefit during the hiking season, but a life-threatening hazard during the summer. A permit is required and may be obtained from the Backcountry Office in the village, or by mail from Grand Canyon National Park, P.O. Box 129, Grand Canyon, Arizona 86023, (928) 638-7888, www.nps.gov/grca.

HOW TO GET THERE Grand Canyon Village is 81 miles north of Flagstaff via U.S. 180 and Arizona 64.

DESCRIPTION The Bright Angel Trailhead is at the west end of the village, and the Boucher Trail starts from Hermit Trailhead at Hermits Rest, at the west end of the West Rim Drive. This one-way hike uses

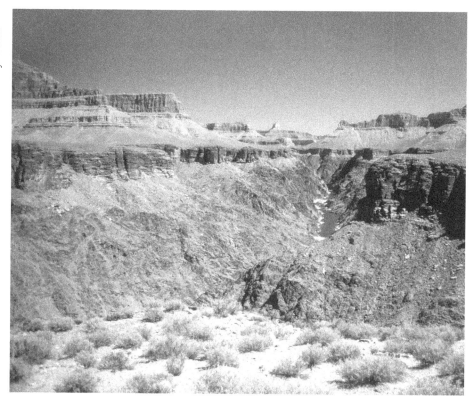

Tonto Trail, Grand Canyon National Park

the Boucher Trail to reach the Tonto Trail, which you follow east along the Tonto Plateau to the Bright Angel Trail and back to the south rim. As Grand Canyon Trails go, the Boucher and this segment of the Tonto Trail are in good shape and are easy to follow. The Bright Angel Trail is a heavily used mule trail.

Roslyn Bullas

28 Highline Trail

RATINGS (1–10)			MILES	DAYS
Scenery	Solitude	Difficulty	42.2	5
6	3	4		

MAPS Pine, Buckhead Mesa, Kehl Ridge, Dane Canyon, Diamond Point, Knoll Lake, Promontory Point, Woods Canyon U.S.G.S.

SEASON April–November.

BEST April–May, September–October.

HIGHLIGHTS This National Recreation Trail, though not a wilderness trail, is a unique hiking experience through Arizona's scenic Mogollon Rim country.

PROBLEMS The Dude Fire burned the central section of the trail in 1990, so you can expect ongoing problems with trail erosion and deadfall.

HOW TO GET THERE The west end of the Highline Trail starts from the Pine Trailhead, which is just south of the village of Pine, on Arizona 87 north of Payson. The east end of the trail meets Arizona Highway 260 at the 260 Trailhead, on Arizona Highway 260 northeast of Payson, on the left just before the Mogollon Rim.

DESCRIPTION The Highline Trail traverses the base of the Mogollon Rim, crossing numerous perennial streams. Several intersecting north-south trails connect to roads south and north of the trail, so you could break the Highline Trail into shorter segments.

29 Apache Railroad Trail

RATINGS (1–10)			MILES	DAYS
Scenery	Solitude	Difficulty	19.1	2
8	2	2		

MAPS Big Lake North, Mount Baldy, Greer, Greens Peak U.S.G.S.

SEASON May–November.

BEST June–October.

HIGHLIGHTS The Apache Railroad Trail follows a section of the old Apache Railroad through the White Mountains and traverses beautiful alpine meadows through the high country. Originally built as a logging railroad, it survived as a tourist railroad until the late 1960s. The U.S. Forest Service, working with volunteer groups, recently constructed a recreation trail along the old railroad grade. The trail is open to horses, mountain bikes, and hikers.

PROBLEMS Roads closely parallel sections of the trail, so don't expect a wilderness experience. Strangely enough, there are few water sources in this otherwise well-watered country. Be sure to pick up enough water for a dry camp when you cross the West Fork of the Little Colorado River, since there's no camping in the immediate area. Other water sources are difficult to reach.

HOW TO GET THERE The south end of the trail starts near Big Lake, which is reached via Arizona 260, Arizona 273, Forest Road 116, and Forest Road 249E. The north trailhead is on Arizona 260.

DESCRIPTION From Big Lake, the Apache Railroad Trail heads north to cross the East and West Forks of the Little Colorado River, just east of the Mount Baldy Wilderness. The trail passes the Sheep Crossing Trailhead, and works its way northwest around several large lakes to end at Arizona 260 near the boundary of the White Mountain Apache Reservation.

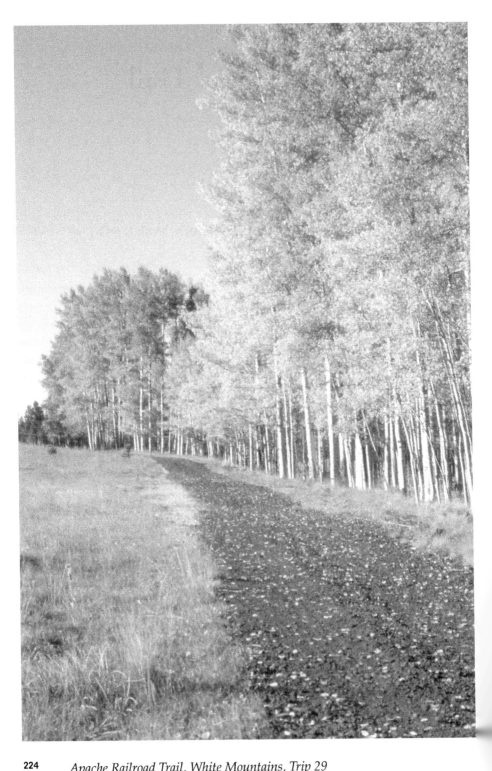

Apache Railroad Trail, White Mountains, Trip 29

30 Sabino–Lemmon Rock Loop

RATINGS (1–10)			MILES	DAYS
Scenery	Solitude	Difficulty	31	4
8	4	6		

MAPS Santa Catalina Mountains Trail and Recreation Map (Rainbow Expeditions)

SEASON March–November.

BEST April–May, September–October.

HIGHLIGHTS The backpacking residents of Tucson are extremely lucky to have two mountain wildernesses right in their back yard. This loop hike follows trails in the Santa Catalina Mountains north of the city, and takes you from Sonoran desert foothills to pine and fir forested mountains and back. It's only one of many possibilities for backpack trips in the Santa Catalina unit of the Coronado National Forest.

PROBLEMS The lower, desert section of this loop is hot during the summer, while the highest elevation may have snow from December through March. In addition, more than 7000 feet of elevation change are involved.

HOW TO GET THERE From Tucson, drive to the north end of Sabino Canyon Road and the Sabino Canyon Visitor Center.

DESCRIPTION From the Sabino Canyon Visitor Center at 2700 feet, follow the Esperero Canyon Trail, the Cathedral Rock Trail, and the Wilderness of Rocks Trail to Lemmon Rock Lookout (8700 feet) near the top of the mountain. Return via the Mount Lemmon Trail, the West Fork Sabino Canyon Trail, and the Bear Canyon Trail.

31 Rincon Crest Loop

RATINGS (1–10)			MILES	DAYS
Scenery	Solitude	Difficulty	35.6	4–5
8	3	6		

MAPS Rincon Mountains (Rainbow Expeditions), Saguaro National Park (Trails Illustrated).

SEASON March–November.

BEST April–May, September–October.

HIGHLIGHTS This loop hike takes you from the desert to the forested summit of the Rincon Mountains, Tucson's other "backyard" mountain range. The Rincon Mountains are one of southern Arizona's classic "sky island" ranges.

Warning: The lower, desert portions of this loop are extremely hot in summer, and the high country may have snow from December through April.

PROBLEMS These trails are within the Rincon Mountain Unit of Saguaro National Park. Because of the park's proximity to the city, the trails are very popular. A permit must be obtained from the park Visitor Center, and camping is allowed at designated backcountry campsites only. Water sources are far apart on this loop.

Tip: Each member of the party should have water capacity for a dry camp.

HOW TO GET THERE From Tuscon, drive east on Broadway, and then south on Old Spanish Trail past the Visitor Center to the Javelina Picnic Area and Trailhead.

DESCRIPTION Start the loop on the Tanque Verde Ridge Trail, which climbs east along its namesake ridge past Juniper Basin, a designated campsite, over Tanque Verde Peak to Cow Head Saddle. The route turns right here, and uses a short connecting trail to reach the Manning Camp Trail, where you turn left and head east once again. At the next trail junction, turn right on a short connecting trail to the Heartbreak Ridge Trail. Turn left and hike north and northwest to the Fire Loop Trail. A right turn here takes you northeast over Man Head and past Reef Rock Fire.

The Fire Loop Trail then turns west and loops over Mica Mountain, the high point of the range at 8664 feet. Continue west past Spud Rock and Helens Dome and down the Cow Head Saddle Trail. At Cow Head Saddle, turn right onto the Douglas Spring Trail, and follow this trail north to Douglas Spring and campsite, and then west along the foothills. A complicated maze of trails covers the northwest corner of the park use the Three Tanks, Pink Hill, and Cactus Forest trails to return to the trailhead.

32 Cave Creek Loop

RATINGS (1–10)			MILES	DAYS
Scenery	Solitude	Difficulty	23.4	3
8	4	6		

MAPS Rustler Park, Chiricahua Peak U.S.G.S.

SEASON May–November.

BEST September–October.

HIGHLIGHTS This loop hike starts from the spectacular Portal area on the east side of the Chiricahua Mountains, climbs to the crest of the range and descends via another trail. It offers some of the best scenery to be found in the Chiricahuas.

PROBLEMS The Chiricahua Mountains have experienced several large wildfires in recent years. Expect problems with erosion and deadfall along some of the trails. Water can be scarce along the Crest Trail section of the route.

HOW TO GET THERE Take Arizona 80 northeast from Douglas, turn left to Portal, and park at the Sunny Flat Campground.

DESCRIPTION Although the first and last couple of miles of the loop are on dirt roads, it's hardly worth bringing a shuttle vehicle to avoid them. Hike south on the road to South Fork Campground, and continue on the South Fork Trail. The route continues on the Burro Trail to Horseshoe Pass and uses the Horseshoe Trail to connect to the south end of the Crest Trail near Sentinel Peak. Follow the Crest Trail north to Cima Park, and head east down Cima Canyon on the Greenhouse Trail. At the junction with the Basin Trail, follow dirt roads past the Southwestern Research Station to Sunny Flat Campground.

Index

S